SURGERY - PROCEDURES, COMPLICATIONS, AND RESULTS

COMBINED STIMULATING METHODS OF RECONSTRUCTIVE SURGERY IN PEDIATRIC ORTHOPEDICS

Surgery - Procedures, Complications, and Results

Additional books in this series can be found on Nova's website under the Series tab.

Additional e-books in this series can be found on Nova's website under the e-book tab.

Surgery - Procedures, Complications, and Results

Combined Stimulating Methods of Reconstructive Surgery in Pediatric Orthopedics

Dmitry Popkov
Editor

New York

NOTICE TO THE READER

Library of Congress Cataloging-in-Publication Data

ISBN: 978-1-63483-028-7
Library of Congress Control Number: 2015940904

Published by Nova Science Publishers, Inc. † New York

CONTENTS

FOREWORD

The Ilizarov method of bone lengthening, reconstruction and osteosynthesis has been developed immensely since its introduction by G.A. Ilizarov in the Soviet Union in the 1960s and in Western countries in the early 1980s. It has become an integral part of the arsenal used by the orthopedic community worldwide. The evolutionary development of the method and its current role has considerably improved the quality of life for millions of people in the whole world.

At the same time, the technology of intramedullary nailing dramatically changed the quality of treatment in tremendous amounts of orthopedic cases. And as we know, brilliant ideas are usually the result of good combinations. Finding this successful meeting point was the goal of Dmitry Popkov and his team! They developed distinguished ideas in deep theoretical, experimental and clinical research within the field of lengthening and deformity correction.

Dr. Popkov et al. found the way to compensate the weakest aspects of Ilizarov techniques by implementing more comfort to patients with a very low chance of complications. Flexible intramedullary nailing improves the stability of the Ilizarov frame with significant decrease in the duration of ExFix. The parts of the book made by Pierre Journeau, Dmitry Popkov and Pierre Lascombes are the unique guidance in treatment of patients with systemic bone diseases and limb length discrepancy with the good analyses of possible problems and complications.

The fundamental research and clinical experience of Professor Arnold Popkov in bone marrow stimulation, using bioactive nailing is another important information which can be used with success in the most challenging group of patients with congenital and genetic bone disorders.

I hope that this valuable information can be used in many challenging orthopedic cases. These great ideas and experimental combinations can really inspire the orthopedic community to better the lives of millions of patients with the most challenging bone disorders.

Alexander Gubin
Ilizarov Center Kurgan CEO,
MD, PhD,
Professor, chair of Orthopedics and Traumatology Tumen Medical Academy,
AOSpine Educational Adviser,
Chief Editor of «The Ilizarov Journal of Clinical and Experimental Orthopedics»

ACKNOWLEDGMENT

I am grateful to my wife Natalia without whom the realization of this book could not have been achieved.

Dmitry Popkov

INTRODUCTION

Dmitry Popkov, PhD, MD

Federal Russian State-Financed Ilizarov Scientific Center for Restorative Traumatology and Orthopaedics, Kurgan, Russia

Methods of surgical treatment in pediatric orthopedics traditionally progress improving implants, external fixation devices, advancing surgical technique, approaches. Comparative studies of various surgical treatment methods, assessment of their advantages and disadvantages are often found in literature. Such approach can undesignedly make a reader consider those methods (for example, external and internal fixation) as contesting, and even worse - to regard them incompatible. However, it is not true.

In this monograph we summarized experience of application of combined methods of surgical deformity correction and limb shortening, spinal deformities in children affected with pathologies when association of external and internal fixation provided quantitative addition of strong points of various osteosynthesis methods, allowed to avoid inconveniencies of each single method as well as achieved qualitative improvement in treatment of complicated pathology of the loco motor system. First of all it is concerned a combined application of Ilizarov method and flexible intramedullary nailing (Nancy method).

Experimental study of that surgical technique and its clinical results are presented in the book. Success of new technologies, of new methods is impossible if natural biologic resources of the body are not involved. It is very important to avoid or reduce negative influence of treatment on the natural growth potential of operated limb segments. It is experimental and clinical study of influence on the growth and limb development after surgery that a part of the monograph is devoted.

Finally, a considerable part of the book concerns application of bioactive implants, influence of micro- and nanosurface on modeling of reparative osteogenesis, it is especially important in systemic skeletal diseases including metabolic osteopathies. The latest innovations of Professor Arnold Popkov and results of their clinical introduction are presented in that chapter.

Reconstructive surgery in pediatric orthopedics described in this book are based on fundamental principles of the Ilizarov method: stability of fixation, preserved bone blood supply, optimal tate and rhythm of distraction, functional limb weight bearing during treatment [1]. However, use of methods of reparative osteogenesis stimulation, limb lengthening by means of combined techniques (external and internal fixation), application of bioactive implants are new directions of Ilizarov method development. Gubin A. et al. consider methods of osteogenesis stimulation as one of prospective research trends [2]. Other important branches of Ilizarov method development are better control of treatment, infection barriers and patient comfort [2].

We greatly appreciate everyone's contribution in writing of this monograph. Hopefully, it will be helpful to specialists involved in management of loco-motor system diseases.

References

Ilizarov GA (1990) Clinical application of the tension *Clin Orthop Relat Res.* 250:8-26.

Gubin AV, Borzunov DY, Malkova TA (2013) *The Ilizarov paradigm: thirty years with the Ilizarov method Int Orthop.* 37(8):1533-1539.

In: Combined Stimulating Methods …
Editor: Dmitry Popkov
ISBN: 978-1-63483-028-7

Chapter I

Limb Lengthening by Combined Technique (External Fixator and Flexible Intramedullary Nailing): Experimental Studies

Dmitry Popkov [*] ***and Arnold Popkov***
Scientific and Clinical Laboratory for Deformity Correction and Limb Lengthening. Federal Russian State-Financed Ilizarov Scientific Center for Restorative Traumatology and Orthopaedics, Kurgan, Russia

Abstract

The experimental results of application of bioinert and bioactive intramedullary nailing in tibial lengthening in mongrels are presented in Chapter I. Basing on data of radiologic, angiographic and morphologic investigations, the advantages of combination of circular external fixation and flexible intramedullary nailing in a gradual limb lengthening are proved from the point of view of stimulation of the osteogenesis and accelerated formation of the distraction regenerate.

Keywords: Combined technique of limb lengthening, experimental study

[*] Corresponding author: Ilizarov Scientific Center for Restorative Traumatology and Orthopaedics, 6, M.-Ulyanova Street, 640014 Kurgan, Russia; dpopkov@mail.ru.

I.1. Tibial Lengthening with Flexible Intramedullary Inert Nailing

Introduction

Based on our extensive experience with the Ilizarov lengthening method, we have demonstrated that one of its fundamentals is preservation of periosteum and intramedullary circulation. Furthermore, quality of the regenerate depends on the lengthening rate, which can be individualized [2]. Automatic high-frequency lengthening and compression of the regenerate immediately after the lengthening period provide optimal conditions for tissue regeneration, and result in significant reduction of the external fixation period [3]. Works have been done to demonstrate the prominent role of periosteum in distraction osteogenesis [4, 5]. Intramedullary nailing provides a strong elastic frame, which enhances the formation of periosteal callus. Additionally, as the two intramedullary nails do not completely fill the medullary cavity, endosteal callus formation is not inhibited. We have worked on the FIN concept to ensure compatibility with the Ilizarov method for limb lengthening. The following study conducted in dogs allows better understanding of our philosophy, and evaluating all the benefits of this combined method.

Materials and Methods

This study was conducted in 14 dogs of various breeds, aged 1 to 4 years, with the average weight of 18.8 kg. The mean length of tibia was 187 mm. The applied Ilizarov fixator consisted of two distal rings and two proximal three-quarter rings, connected by threaded rods. Both, percutaneous osteotomy of the fibula and osteoclasis of the tibia were performed in the middle third of the diaphysis. The FIN construct used two 1.5 mm nails with opposing curves (Figure 1). Both nails were sharply contoured, and their tips bent to 30–40° over a length of 2–3 mm. Their initial curves were identical, with apex located in the midsection. Both nails had blunt tips. Two slightly oblique entry holes were made with an awl in the superior portion of the proximal metaphysis. The first nail was hand pushed into the medullary canal, then across the osteoclasis and down to the distal metaphysis, as far as possible into the cancellous bone. The second nail was inserted in the same manner, on the opposite side of the bone. The final construct consisted of two nails with opposing curves positioned in the same plane. The free ends (trailing ends) of the nails were cut relatively short and bent to about 45–60° to prevent nail migration during distraction. The skin was closed in one layer. Distraction was initiated on the fifth day in all dogs (Figure 1). Duration of lengthening was 28 days. Mean distraction rate was 1 mm/day (in four steps) (Table I.1.1).

However, as control X-rays showed extensive bone regenerate, the distraction speed had to be increased on D 8 in 4 dogs, D 15 in 3, and D 21 in 1. Early healing occurred twice in about 21 days of lengthening, and twice in about 28 days: in two cases, distraction resulted in fracture of the regenerate that had already consolidated (Figure 2), whereas in the other two cases, the newly regenerated bone was already very strong. The 28-day lengthening period was followed by the external fixation period. The external fixator was removed after 15 days (sixth week) in eight dogs and 30 days (eighth week) in four. All the dogs could bear weight right after removal of the external fixator without any limb protection.

Table I.1.1. Duration of the lengthening and external fixation

Period	Osteoclasis, Ilizarov +FIN	Distraction (lengthening)	External fixation	Removal of external fixation
Date	Day 0	Days 5-33	Days 34-49=6 dogs Days 34-63=8 dogs	Days 49=6 dogs Day 63=8 dogs

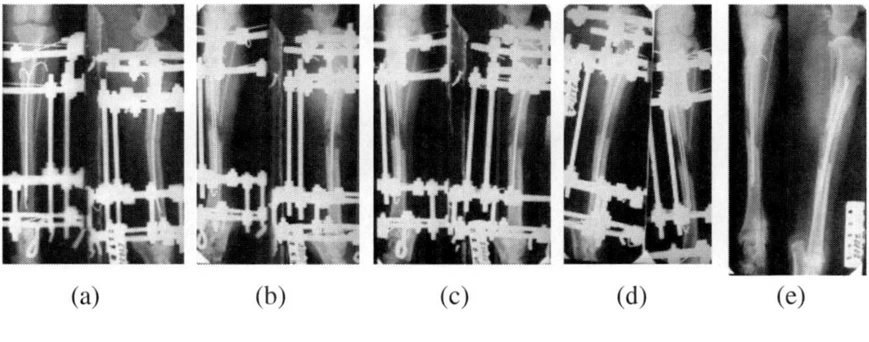

(a) (b) (c) (d) (e)

Figure 1. Radiograph of the right tibia. Tibial lengthening by combined Ilizarov/FIN: Ilizarov fixator and intramedullary nails in place, osteoclasis of the tibia(a); X-ray taken after 21 days of lengthening(b); X-ray taken after 28 days of lengthening (end of lengthening period) (c). Note the intense and extensive periosteal reaction, and a growth zone with numerous bone trabeculae. Thirty millimeter lengthening: Complete healing achieved after 14 days of external fixation (d); external fixator removed (e); X-ray taken 15 days (D 63) after removal of the external fixator and resumption of weight bearing.

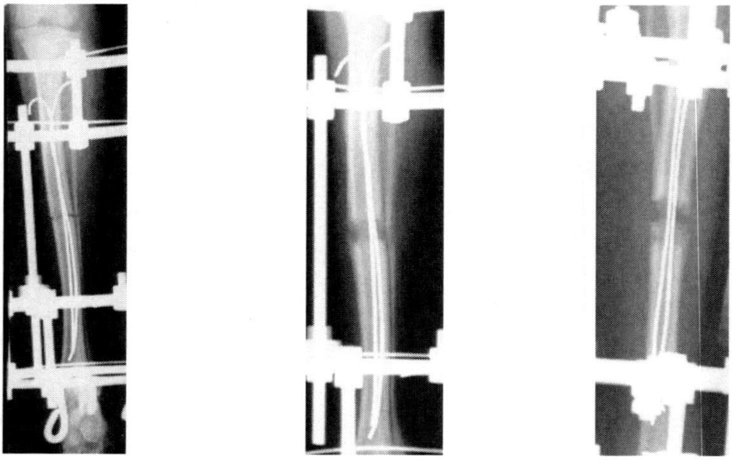

(a) (b) (c)

Figure 2. Healing status after 14 days of tibial lengthening using combined Ilizarov/FIN: Ilizarov fixator and two intramedullary nails in place, closed osteoclasis of the tibia (a); X-ray taken after 14 days of lengthening at a rate of 1.75 mm/day (b); X-ray taken after 21 days of lengthening, fracture of the regenerate (c).

Results were evaluated according to the radiographic appearance of the regenerate. Control X-rays were performed on a weekly basis throughout the distraction period, and thereafter, at 45 days, 60 days, and after removal of the intramedullary nails. Arteriographies were performed in some dogs after sacrifice: at D 5, 39, and 63. Additionally, bone regenerates were histologically studied.

Results

Radiological changes proved intense and extensive bone regeneration, it forced us to increase the distraction speed in some dogs. Newly formed bone was visible on radiographs after 7 days of lengthening. At this stage, the regenerate had an inhomogeneous structure with localized areas of increased bone density. Extensive periosteal reaction (21.6 mm long, 0.5–2.0 mm thick) could be noted along the bone fragments. At 2 weeks, the regenerate was well structured and filled completely the interfragmentary gap. The growth zone contained numerous bone trabeculae. Periosteal reaction was 24–26 mm long and 2–3 mm thick. The regenerate was larger than the tibia. In 15 days of fixation (D 48), the regenerate was completely consolidated in all the animals. Cortical bone was reconstructed. Continuity of three or four cortices was reestablished along the regenerate. The growth zone had disappeared. A denser periosteal reaction was noted. In 30 days of fixation (D 63), the medullary canal was already formed in three out of four dogs. No fracture or deformity occurred after removal of the external fixator because the regenerates had already consolidated, and also because the bones were protected by FIN.

After 15 days of external fixation, histology showed cortical continuity, fully interconnected cancellous trabeculae, and disappearance of the fibrous layer surrounding the new bone (Figure 3a). As a matter of fact, consolidation took place during the fixation period and lasted 2 weeks.

Thirty days after removal of the external fixator, the cortices were thicker. Remodeling of the medullary canal was under way. We were happy to note extensive tissue regeneration along the intramedullary nail (Figure 3b).

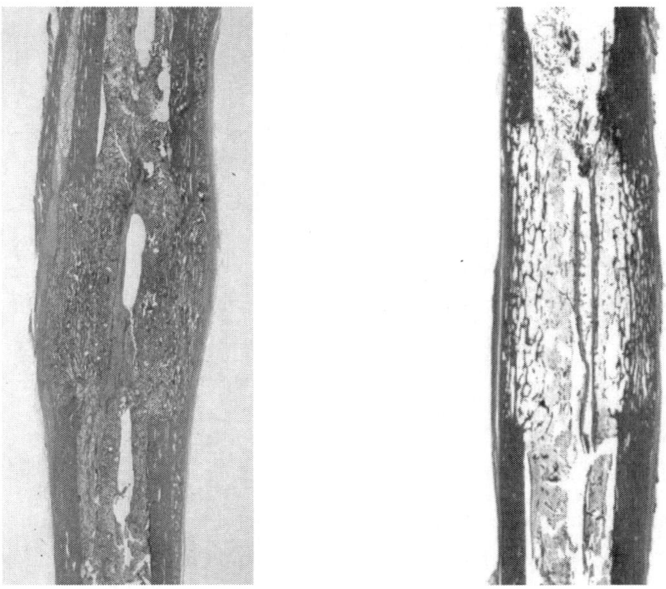

(a) (b)

Figure 3. Histologic sections (tibia): specimen at D 49 (fixator removed), cortices were present along the regenerate and continuity was re-established. Growth zone was no longer visible (a); specimen at D 88, 25 days after removal of the external fixator, intramedullary nails were removed just before sacrifice (b). Regenerate consisted of cortical and cancellous bone tissue. The medullary canal was patent. Ossification was present along the intramedullary nails.

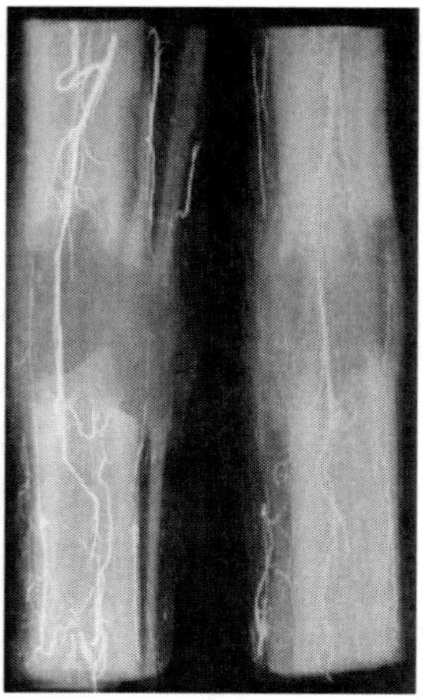

(a)

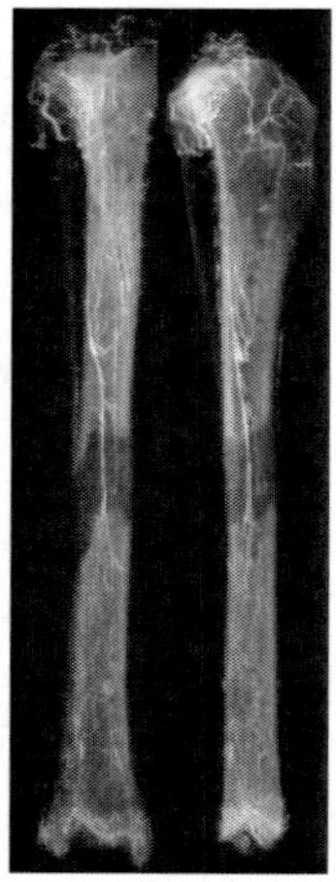

(b)

Figure 4. Arteriography: the medullary artery was patent (tibia-dog): Arteriography (AP and lateral) of specimen after removal of the intramedullary nails on the 6th day of the fixation period (D 39) (a); arteriography (AP and lateral) after 30 days of fixation (D 63) (b).

This structure can be compared to a stainless steel lead pencil.

Arteriographies performed at the initiation of lengthening, after 6 days of external fixation, and immediately after removal of the intramedullary nails (Figure 4), showed that the medullary artery had remained patent all the time.

No implant migration or skin problems occurred. We found that proper nail contouring ensured stability of bone fragments during lengthening.

Discussion

The Ilizarov lengthening method has revolutionized the biology of bone and bone growth. Preservation of bone environment, periosteum, and particularly, the medullary vascularization, respect of the biological rate of bone growth, use of automatic high-frequency lengthening, preservation of stability and elasticity (provided by the rings): everything works together to provide good to excellent tissue regeneration [3]. The more stable the lengthening site is, the faster it will heal. Though Professor Ilizarov claimed the major role of the bone marrow in new bone formation, a certain number of works disputed the paramount qualitative role of periosteum in distraction osteogenesis [4, 5].

FIN has a proven track record of over 25 years of effective fracture treatment in children based on animal experimentation [1] and above all, on the outstanding experience of the Pediatric Orthopedic Department, Surgical Clinic, Nancy (France). According to data, FIN builds a strong elastic frame that enhances biological effect of redistribution of blood flow to the periosteal structures through cortical canals, thus stimulating formation of periosteal callus. FIN is a semi-rigid elastic nailing system, that allows cyclic micro-scale plastic deformations which is most beneficial for healing. Also, as the two intramedullary nails do not fill in the medullary cavity completely, endosteal callus formation is not inhibited.

We had the idea to combine both elastic systems, Ilizarov and FIN, for limb lengthening [6]. Our animal experiments prove that contoured intramedullary nails do not inhibit endosteal bone formation. On the contrary, despite partial destruction of the bone marrow, the preserved intramedullary circulation stimulates tissue regeneration to such an extent that it becomes necessary to increase the distraction speed to avoid premature consolidation of the regenerate during lengthening.

The biological effect of redistribution of intramedullary blood flow to the periosteal structures stimulates formation of periosteal callus, resulting in extensive periosteal reaction, both along the bone fragments and at the diastasis. FIN provides increased stability at the diastasis by resisting translation motion (essentially) in the plane of the nails. Gradual stretching or sliding of the intramedullary nails through the regenerate during lengthening seems to enhance the regeneration process. However, the mechanism of biological stimulation of endosteal bone formation remains unexplained. Controlled bone marrow irritation by an intramedullary nail is known to produce localized new bone formation [1]. It has been confirmed in animals, when intramedullary nails positioned at the periphery of the regenerate and gradually pulled have shown to accelerate the formation of new bone [7].

Conclusion

FIN can be used together with external fixation for bone lengthening. Combined use of these two methods allows to stimulate both endosteal and periosteal bone formation. FIN improves stability of the bone fragments at the diastasis, and does not inhibit intramedullary circulation. In bone lengthening, FIN is the only internal fixation method that provides the same optimal conditions for bone regeneration as the Ilizarov method. That is why combined

Ilizarov/FIN yields such a good outcome. The results of this experimental study have been, in our Kurgan clinic, a determining factor for the use of combined Ilizarov/FIN method in bone lengthening and correction of bone deformities in patients with limb length discrepancy (LLD) and skeletal pathologies such as hereditary hypophosphatemic rickets.

I.2. Tibial Lengthening with Flexible Intramedullary Nailing with Hydroxyapatite Coating

As mentioned in the previous chapter, the combined technique of lengthening (external fixator+FIN) boosts bone consolidation. Obviously, it is provided by mechanical peculiarities of osteosynthesis: increase of stability of bone fragments and gradual traction of intramedullary nails along the medullary cavity. This effect manifests only if the intramedullary blood supply is preserved – a fundamental condition of the Ilizarov method.

It is well-known that implants with hydroxyapatite coating, like prosthetic stems, have better adhesion with bone tissue because of biologic reaction of bone formation immediately on the implant without an intermediate fibrous layer. In other words, surfaces of such implants reveal osteoconductive features [8-12].

We held an experiment in dogs, when nails covered with hydroxyapatite were inserted in the medullary canal for tibial lengthening by the combined technique.

The results are presented in this chapter.

Materials and Methods

This study was conducted in 12 dogs of various breeds, aged from 1 to 4 years, with the average weight of 18.2 kg. The mean length of tibia was 181 mm. The applied Ilizarov fixator consisted of two distal rings and two proximal three-quarter rings, connected by threaded rods (Figure5). The only difference from the series with bioinert intramedullary nails described in the previous chapter was application of lesser number of wires in the Ilizarov fixator. The upper and lower systems contained only three wires each. There was no other difference between the surgical techniques.

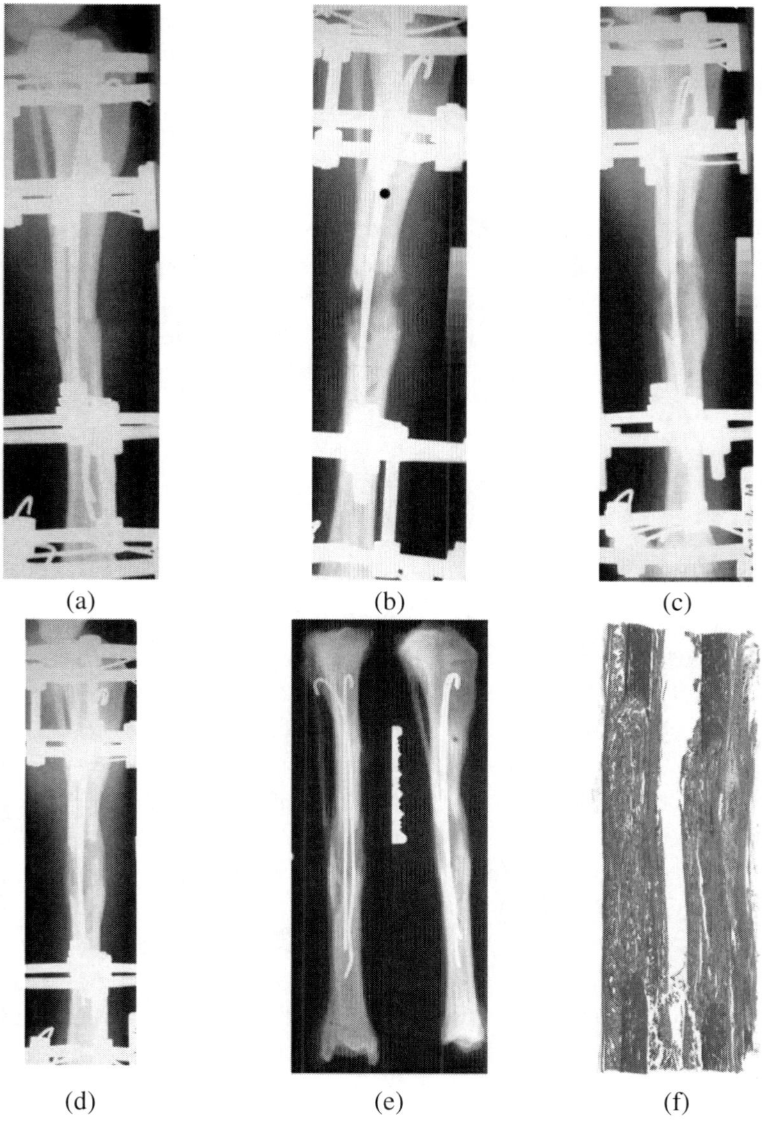

Figure 5. Radiograph of the *right tibia*. Tibial lengthening by combined Ilizarov/FIN: Ilizarov fixator and intramedullary nails in place, osteoclasis of the tibia(**a**); X-ray taken after 28 days of lengthening (end of lengthening period) (**b**); X-ray taken after 7 days (D 40) of fixation period (**c**). Complete healing achieved after 14 days of fixation period (D 48)(**d**); external fixator removed (**e**). Histologic sections (tibia): specimen at D 49 (fixator removed), cortices were present along the regenerate and continuity was re-established.

Distraction was initiated on the fifth day in all dogs (Figure 5). The mean distraction rate at the beginning was 1 mm/day. Duration of lengthening was 28 days. A 28-day- lengthening period was followed by external fixation period. The external fixator was removed after 15 days of fixation (D 48) in all dogs. All the dogs could bear weight right after removal of the external fixator without any limb protection.

Results were evaluated according to the radiographic appearance of the regenerate. X-ray control was performed weekly throughout the distraction and fixation periods and after frame removal. Additionally, bone regenerates were histologically studied after sacrifice: at D 48 and D 63.

Results

As in the first series, radiological changes indicated intense and extensive bone regeneration, that forced us to increase the distraction speed in some dogs. Newly formed bone was visible on radiographs after D 7 of lengthening. At this stage, the regenerate had an inhomogeneous structure with localized areas of increased bone density. An intensive periosteal reaction (15–54 mm long and 3-10 mm thick) developed by the 2nd-3rd week of distraction period. It caused significant enlargement of bone cross-sectional dimensions (Figure 6).

As control X-rays revealed extensive bone regenerate, the distraction speed had to be increased in 7 dogs. Early healing occurred in four dogs by the 14th-21st day of lengthening. The following lengthening did not resulted in rupture of the regenerate that had already consolidated (Figure 7). After 15 days of fixation (D 48), the regenerate was completely healed in all the animals. Cortical bone was reconstructed. Continuity of three or four cortices was reestablished along the regenerate. The growth zone had disappeared. A denser periosteal reaction was noted. No fracture or deformity occurred after removal of the external fixator because the regenerates had already consolidated, besides the bones were protected by FIN.

At the same time, a histological study showed cortical continuity, fully interconnected cancellous trabeculae and disappearance of the fibrous layer surrounding the new bone (Figure 5f, 6e). In fact, consolidation happened during the fixation period and lasted 2 weeks. Similar to bioinert intramedullary nails, the extensive tissue regeneration along the intramedullary nail was noted (Figure 5f, 6e).

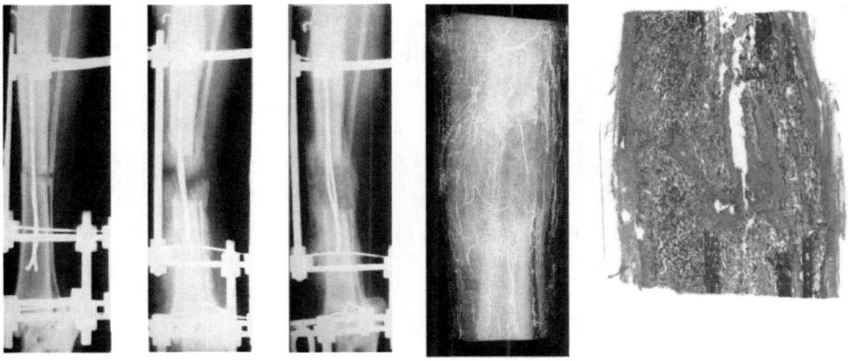

(a) (b) (c) (d) (e)

Figure 6. Intensive periosteal reaction: Ilizarov fixator and intramedullary nails in place, osteoclasis of the tibia(**a**); by the end of distraction (D 33) an intensive periosteal reaction developed at a level of the gap and adjacent bone fragments (**b**); bone consolidation was defined in two weeks of fixation (D 47), bone diameter doubled at a level of lengthening (**c**); arteriography by the sacrifice revealed a significant osteogenesis in periosteal and endosteal parts of new bone (**d**). Histologic sections: specimen at D 49 (fixator removed), cortices were present along the regenerate and continuity was re-established. Regenerate consisted of cortical and cancellous bone tissue. The medullary canal was patent. Ossification was present along the intramedullary nails. Periosteal reaction resulted in doubled bone diameter at a level of lengthening. (**e**).

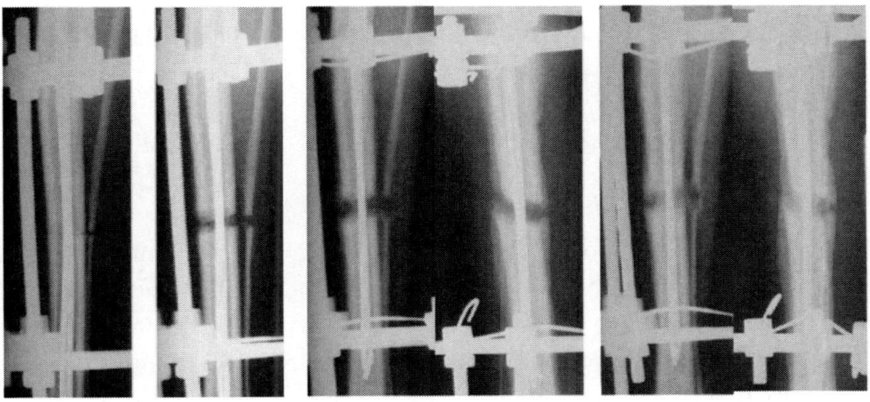

(a) (b) (c) (d)

Figure 7. Healing status after 14 days of tibial lengthening using combined Ilizarov/FIN: Ilizarov fixator and two intramedullary nails in place, closed osteoclasis of the tibia (**a**); X-ray taken after 7 days of lengthening (**b**); X-ray taken after 14 days of lengthening, the gap size did not correspond to the duration of distraction, the bone regenerate is uninterrupted, a continued periosteal reaction at the level of lengthening and bone fragments - consolidation (**c**); X-ray taken after 28 days of lengthening, no separation of bone fragments (the gap did not increased), wires of the Ilizarov fixator did not gain in curve, the regenerate did not ruptured (**d**).

Arteriographies, performed immediately after removal of the intramedullary nails (Figure 6d), showed exuberant formation of the vascular net in the regenerate and periosteal structures.

Besides, no implant migration, septic complications, secondary displacement of bone fragments or skin problems were observed. An ensured stability of bone fragments during lengthening was noted applying the flexible intramedullary nails with hydroxyapatite coating even if the number of wires in the Ilizarov frame was diminished.

Discussion

Preservation of bone environment, periosteum and, particularly, the medullary vascularization, respect of the biological rate of bone growth, preservation of stability and elasticity (provided by the rings) - all these work together to ensure excellent tissue regeneration [13,14].

Our previous animal experiments prove that contoured titanium intramedullary nails do not inhibit endosteal bone formation. On the contrary, despite partial destruction of the bone marrow, the preserved intramedullary circulation stimulates tissue regeneration.

Mechanical impact of gradual traction of flexible nails in the medullar cavity and increased stability at the diastasis by resisting translation motion (essentially) in the plane of the nails as demonstrated before [14] induce stimulation of the regeneration process.

The added bioactive intramedullary element in this situation appeared to to increase a favorable effect of the FIN.

Hydroxyapatite-coated intramedullary nails were chosen because of osteoconductive features of this mineral [15,16]. The fact of solid adhesion between bone and hydroxyapatite implants [8,9,12] was proved. Hydroxyapatite coating provides an early fixation of an implant without a fibrous layer between bone and implant. Soballe et al. [17] demonstrated that the fibrous tissue beneath HA interface contains collagen fibers which are usually perpendicular to the implant surface and can guide bony ongrowth.

Hydroxyapatite-coated intramedullary nails used in the experiment intensified formation of bone distraction regenerate. It ensured consolidation of bone fragments within two weeks after the end of distraction in all cases. The combined technique of distraction osteosynthesis with bioactive implants was performed with a lightened variant of the external osteosynthesis (fewer wires in the Ilizarov fixator).

We believe that use of hydroxyapatite-coated intramedullary nails in combination with external fixation can be indicated in systemic skeletal diseases, associated with disorders of bone tissue formation, impaired metabolism of Ca and P resulted in low bone mineral density.

Thus, the combined technique of lengthening with bioactive intramedullary implants respects all the favorable aspects of mechanical stimulation of bone formation. The use of hydroxyapatite-coated intramedullary nails allows to decrease the number of wires or half-pins of the external fixator with no harm to stability of osteosynthesis. Besides, the bone healing is achieved in the shortest period.

REFERENCES

[1] Téot, L. (1987). L'enclouage centromédullaire élastique stable chez l'enfant. Cahier d'enseignement de la SOFCOT no 28. Expansion Scientifique Française, Paris, 71–90.

[2] Lascombes, P., Membre, H., Prévot, J. & Barat, E. (1991). Histomorphométrie du régénérat osseux dans les allongements des membres selon la technique d'Ilizarov. *Rev Chir Orthop.*, *77*, 141–150.

[3] Shevtsov, V. I., Popkov, A. V., Popkov, D. A. & Prévot, J. (2001). Réduction de la durée du traitement dans les allongements osseux progressifs. *Rev Chir Orthop.*, *87*, 248–256.

[4] Kojimoto, H., Yasui, N., Goto, T., Matsuda, S. & Shimomura, Y. (1988). Bone lengthening by callus distraction. The role of periosteum and endosteum. *J Bone Joint Surg.*, *70B*, 543–549.

[5] Yasui, N., Kojimoto, H., Sasaki, K., Shimizu, H. & Shimomura, Y. (1991). The effects of distraction upon bone, muscle and periosteum. *Orthop Clin North Am.*, *22*, 563–567.

[6] Shevtsov, V. I., Popkov, A. V., Popkov, D. A., Yerofeev, S. A., Prévot, J. & Lascombes, P. (2004). Embrochage centromédullaire dans les allongements osseux selon Ilizarov. *Rev Chir Orthop.*, *90*, 399–410.

[7] Launay, F., Jouve, J. L., Guillaume, J. M., Viehweger, E., Jacquemier, M. & Bollini, G. (2001). Les allongements progressifs de l'avantbras chez l'enfant. À propos d'une série de 14 cas. *Rev Chir Orthop.*, *87*, 786–795.

[8] Dumbleton, J. & Manley, M. T. (2004). Hydroxyapatite-coated prostheses in total hip and knee arthroplasty. *J Bone Joint Surg (Am)*, *86-A*, 2526-2540.

[9] Chatelet, J-C. & Setiey, L. (2004). Comportement osseux à long terme après implantation d'un pivot fémoral totalement revêtu d'hydroxyapatite. *Rev Chir Orthop*, *90*, 628-635.

[10] Kold, S., Rahbek, O., Zippor, B., Bechtold, J. E. & Søballe, K. (2005). Bone compaction enhances fixation of hydroxyapatite-coated implants in a canine gap model. *J Biomed Mater Res B Appl Biomater.*, *75*(1), 49-55.

[11] Rahbek, O., Kold, S., Bendix, K., Overgaard, S. & Søballe, K. (2005). Superior sealing effect of hydroxyapatite in porous-coated implants: experimental studies on the migration of polyethylene particles around stable and unstable implants in dogs. *Acta Orthop*, *76*(3), 375-385.

[12] Epinette, J. A. & Manley, M. T. (2007). Hydroxyapatite-coated total knee replacement: clinical experience at 10 to 15 years. *J Bone Joint Surg Br*, *89*(1), 34-38.

[13] Shevtsov, V. I., Popkov, A. V., Popkov, D. A. & Prévot, J. (2001). Réduction de la durée du traitement dans les allongements osseux progressifs. *Rev Chir Orthop*, *87*, 248–256.

[14] Popkov D., Popkov A., Haumont T., Journeau P. & Lascombes P. (2010). Flexible intramedullary nail use in limb lengthening. *J Pediatr Orthop*, *30*(8), 910-918.

[15] Hacking, S. A., Tanzer, M., Harvey, E. J., Krygier, J. J. & Bobyn, J. D. (2002). Relative contributions of chemistry and topography to the osseointegration of hydroxyapatite coatings. *Clin Orthop Relat Res*, *405*, 24-38.

[16] Popkov, A. V. & Popkov, D. A. (2012). Bioactive implants in traumatology and orthopaedics. *Irkutsk: SCRRS SB RAMS.*, 438 p.

[17] Soballe, K., Hansen, E. S., Rasmussen, H. B. & Bunger, C. (1995) Fixation of porous coated versus HA coated implants. In: Epinette J-A: Geesink RGT: eds. *Hydroxyapatite coated hip and knee arthroplasty.* Vol *51*. Paris: Expansion Scientifique Francaise.

In: Combined Stimulating Methods …
Editor: Dmitry Popkov

ISBN: 978-1-63483-028-7

Chapter II

Influence of the Transphyseal Sliding Nailing on Longitudinal Growth of the Tibia: Experimental Studies

Dmitry Popkov [1*]***, Natalia Kononovich***[1]***,***
Roman Shutov[1] ***and Dominique Barbier***[2]
[1]Scientific and Clinical Laboratory for Deformity Correction and Limb Lengthening. Federal Russian State-Financed Ilizarov Scientific Center for Restorative Traumatology and Orthopaedics, Kurgan, Russia
[2]Pediatric Orthopedic Surgery Dept, Nancy University Hospital Center, Children's Hospital, Vandoeuvre, France

Abstract

Transphyseal sliding nailing of the right intact tibia with thin steel rods was performed in six mongrel dogs at the age of six months. The contralateral segment served as a control. In series II the transphyseal sliding nailing was performed in a fractured tibia also in six dogs. Modifications of residual growth and natural shape-formation of proximal and distal epiphyses of the tibia were observed in the experiment in conditions influenced by the transphyseal rods.

* Corresponding author: Ilizarov Scientific Center for Restorative Traumatology and Orthopaedics, 6, M.-Ulyanova Street, 640014 Kurgan, Russia; dpopkov@mail.ru.

Keywords: Growth, tibia, transphyseal sliding nailing

INTRODUCTION

Skeletal systemic diseases inhibiting strength properties of bone tissue, osteogenesis imperfecta in particular, are very often complicated by pathological fractures, deformities and limb length discrepancy. In 1952, Sofield proposed to perform transphyseal intramedullary reinforcement in order to correct deformities in osteogenesis imperfecta [1]. In this case, intramedullary material stay inside for the whole period of growth serving as an internal device during bone fragment union, as well as preventing the development of new deformities. Further development of the technique of transphyseal reinforcement allowed Bayley to create a specific system of transphyseal intramedullary telescopic osteosynthesis [2-6]. In 1987 Métaizeau proposed to use intramedullary sliding transphyseal elastic nailing not only for treatment of common shaft fractures in children, but also to prevent deformities in skeletal systemic diseases accompanied by bone tissue fragility [7].

There are many recent publications which highlight advantages of the telescopic intramedullary transphyseal systems in prevention of fractures and deformities in children affected with osteogenesis imperfecta [8-10]. In 2004, Boutaud and Laville reported fewer complications comparing to use of telescopic rods in their study of intramedullary transphyseal sliding reinforcement in 14 children with osteogenesis imperfecta (36 segments) [11]. Another advantage of elastic nails is a possibility of applying in any medullary canal diameter that is particularly important for children up to the age of 6 years.

As Salter and Harris demonstrated, the growth cartilage is known to be one of the most important anatomic structures in pediatric orthopedic practice [12]. However, there is no clinical or experimental research of the effect of prolonged transphyseal reinforcement with elastic nails on the growth of involved segment.

Thus, the purpose of this study was to evaluate the influence of transphyseal elastic nailing on the residual growth of intact tibia (series I) or on the tibia with transverse shaft fracture (series II).

Materials and Methods

Experiments were performed observing 12 mongrel dogs in the period of growth (at the age of six months). The animals were divided in two experimental series (six animals in each). Littermate puppies were used in each separate series. Preoperative X-ray examination confirmed the presence of open tibial proximal and distal growth plates in all the dogs.

The sliding bipolar transphyseal elastic intramedullary nailing of the right intact tibia was performed in the first series (Figure 8) [13]. The left limb served as a control.

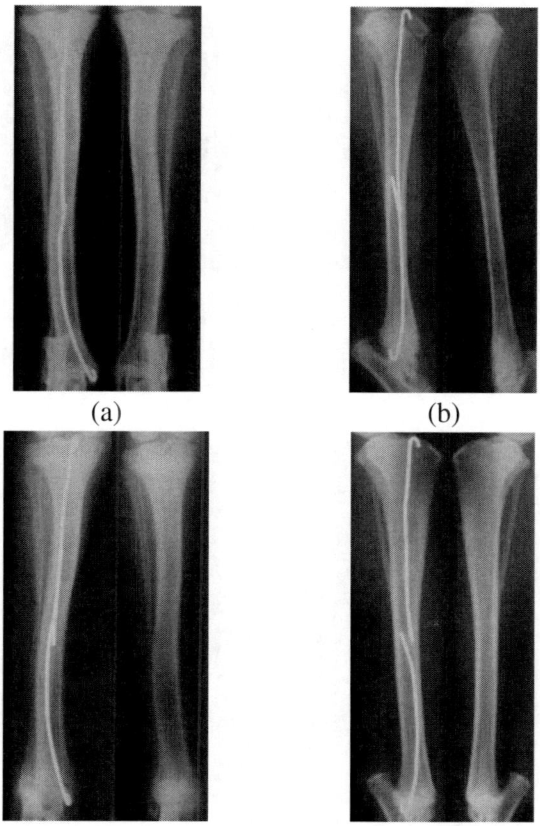

(a) (b)

(c) (d)

Figure 8. Series I: X-rays (D 0, AP view) of the right and left tibiae (**a**); X-rays (D 0, lateral view) of the right and left tibiae (**b**); X-rays (M 6, AP view) of the right and left tibiae (**c**); X-rays (M 6, lateral view) of the right and left tibiae (**d**).

Protocol of surgery. Thiopental intravenous anesthesia was used for all the interventions. A proximal titanium nail of 1.8 mm of diameter and 10 cm in length, pre-curved at 40° was inserted from the approach of 2 cm medially to the proper patellar ligament. Preliminarily, an entry hole towards the medullary canal transphyseally by a single maneuver uwith a surgical awl of 3-mm diameter in the position of the knee flexion. It is through this channel the bent nail was inserted.

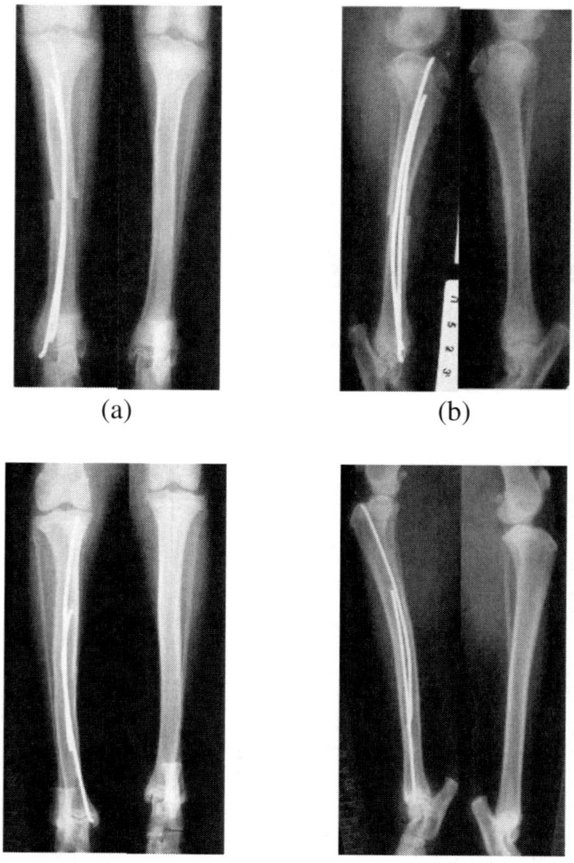

(a) (b)

(c) (d)

Figure 9. Series II: X-rays (D 0, AP view) of the right and left tibiae (**a**); X-rays (D 0, lateral view) of the right and left tibiae (**b**); X-rays (M 6, AP view) of the right and left tibiae (**c**); X-rays (M 6, lateral view) of the right and left tibiae (**d**).

A distal nail was inserted retrogradely at the level of medial malleolus also transphyseally. Free ends of the nails were U-bent and impacted into epiphyses in order to prevent their migration inside the bone during residual growth of the segment. Wounds sutured by layers with interrupted stitches. Thus, preventive intramedullary transphyseal osteosynthesis applied for osteogenesis imperfecta was simulated in this series.

In the second series a transverse osteotomy was performed subperiosteally with a vibro-saw at the level of middle third of the tibial shaft from 2-cm antero-internal approach before insertion of intramedullary titanium nails (Figure 9). Fibular shaft integrity was broken by transcutaneous osteotomy with a chisel. The technique of intramedullary nail insertion was similar to those of the first series, however, the nails were inserted along the entire length of the medullary canal. Thus, in this series intramedullary transphyseal elastic nailing was simulated for pathologic bone fracture in osteogenesis imperfecta.

Postoperative wounds were systematically treated in the postoperative period. The animals were anesthetized using non-steroid anti-inflammatory preparations during the first three days twice a day. Additional immobilization of the operated limb was not performed. The animals moved with full weight-bearing of the operated limb without limitation.

The growth of leg bones in created conditions was studied according to X-ray examination of both legs in AP and lateral views. X-rays were taken on the day of surgery and then once a month for six months (up to the closure of tibial growth plates). Radiography was performed at standard focal distance secureing the examined limb with "VEP X Technology Premium VET" radiological device.

The following parameters were evaluated monthly:

- tibial length was measured by X-rays in the lateral projection of segment axis from tibial condylar articular surface to the ankle gap. The change in tibial length was calculated, as well as the growth length loss comparing with the left tibia (mm and %), the growth for the observation period of the segment final length, and the relative loss of length comparing with the left tibia;
- the amount of crossing of the proximal and distal nails in the medullary canal;

- the diameter of tibial shaft in the middle third (by AP and lateral views of X-rays);
- the mechanical Medial Proximal Tibial Angle (mMPTA) was measured between the mechanical axis of segment and the line connecting two points (tops) of the concave articular surfaces of tibial condyles;
- the mechanical Lateral Distal Tibial Aangle (mLDTA) formed by the mechanical axis of segment and the ankle articular line;
- the location of elastic nails at the level of physes relative to their median axes in the sagittal and frontal planes.

Moreover, in series II the time of bone fragment consolidation was evaluated, as well as possible segment deformities resulted from secondary displacement. Statistical analysis included descriptive statistics: mean values (M) and standard deviation (SD). Comparative studies were carried out with Student's t-test and Wilcoxon test for independent and paired samples. Differences in values considered significant at $p<0.05$. AtteStat 13.1 Program was used to calculate the statistical parameters.

Comparing values within the series were as follows:

- D 0 (day of surgery) vs M 6 (six months after the experiment start) for the right limb,
- D 0 (day of surgery) vs M 6 (six months after the experiment start) for the left limb,
- D 0, the right limb, vs D 0, the left limb,
- M 6, the right limb, vs M 6, the left limb,

The experiments were made in accordance with the requirements of “European Convention for the protection of vertebrate animals used for experimental and other scientific purposes”, and it was approved by Ethics Committee of the Ilizarov Center.

RESULTS

No infectious and neurological complications were observed in any case. Additional surgeries were not required. In all cases the puppies began moving with full weight-bearing of the operated limb in 2-3 days after surgery.

The position of nails relative to physes centers in each series is illustrated in Figure 10. The passage of the nails at the level of distal growth plate was markedly medial due to their insertion through medial malleolus. The nail occupied 0.63±0.03% of metaphysis area in this zone.

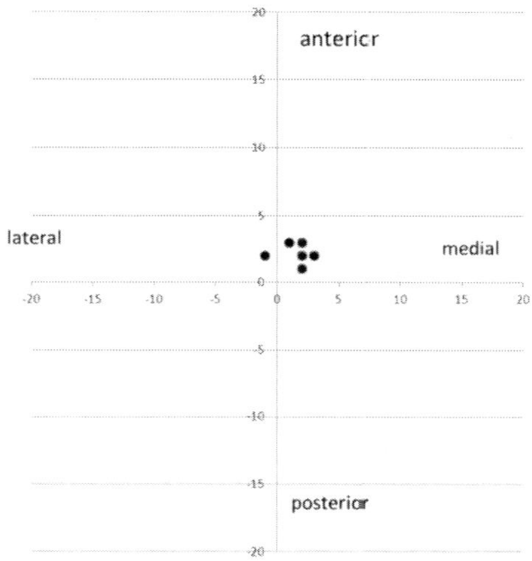

(a)

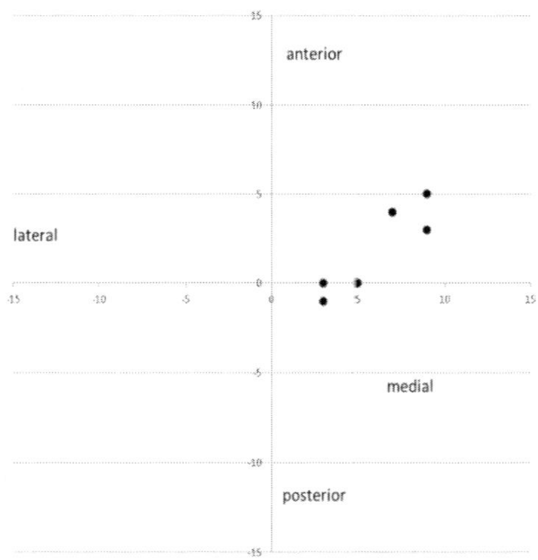

(b)

Figure 10. (Continued).

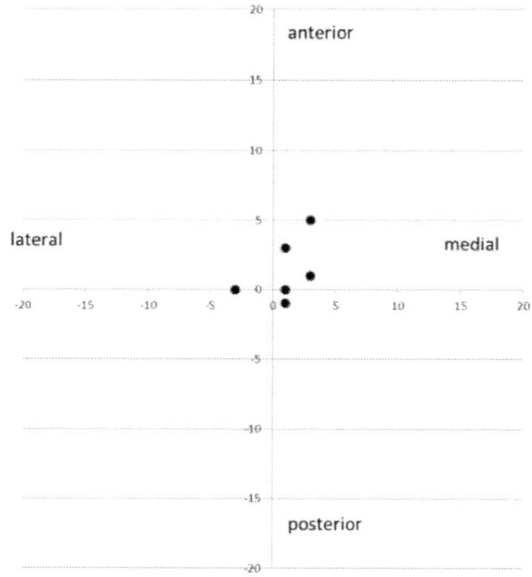

(c)

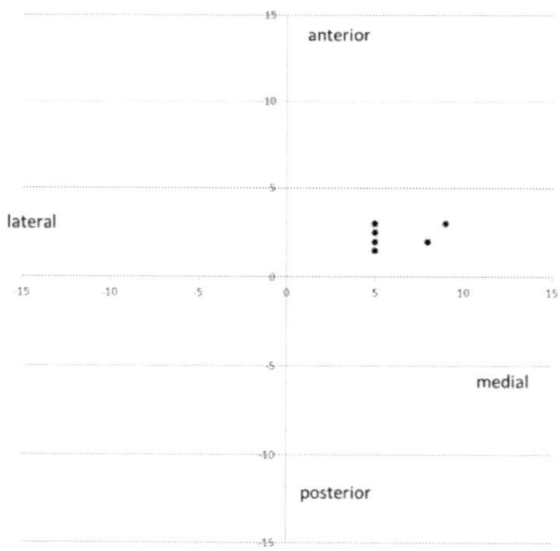

(d)

Figure 10. Location of elastic nails at the level of physes relative to their median axes in the sagittal and frontal planes: proximal tibial physis, series I (**a**); distal tibial physis, series I (**b**); proximal tibial physis, series II (**c**); distal tibial physis, series II (**d**).

At the level of proximal physis the position of the nails was more central, but also, in most cases, with a tendency to 1-5-mm displacement in the medial direction with respect to bone longitudinal axis. The nail occupied 0.32±0.03% of the area of proximal metaphysis. The analysis of the tibial residual growth demonstrated in Table II.1.

As seen from the data, the growth continued in the dogs of all series. Difference between the initial length and the length of tibiae (of the right and left limbs) by the end of the experiment are statistically significant in all the series. However, a smaller longitudinal increase of the operated tibia is also characteristic for the both series of the experiment, but they are not statistically significant. The value of longitudinal growth loss during the experiment is the least. Itamounted to 1-7 mm (from 1 to 5.4%) in series I and from 5 to 17 mm (from 2.8 to 9.5%) in series II, but the growth acceleration of the operated leg was observed in one dog, and the difference in length by the end of the experiment amounted to 5 mm (2.7%).

When analyzing directly the value of tibial gain for D 0 - M 6 period in all the series, a 15-18% decrease of this parameter in the operated segment was determined comparing with the control one.

When measuring the extent of overlapping of nails in the medullary canal, it progressively decreased only as long as the tibia grew. In average the decrease of crossing was 13.4±0.9 mm in the first seriesand 15.6±5.7 mm in the second series by the end of the experiment. There was no significant difference between the series. Migration of the proximal nail inside the bone should be mentioned in two cases of 19 mm and 25 mm in series II. We did not observe the cases of nail inward migration during segment growth in series I.

No reliable differences in mMPTA values of the experimental segment were revealed between themselves and comparing with the preoperative level at different stages of the experiment (Table II.2). Slightly marked changes of this value were found in the left (control) segment. However, these changes were statistically doubtful regarding the experimental segment in four cases. Apparently, the transphyseal insertion of elastic nails close to the center of growth plate doesn't significantly influence the mMPTA value.

Table II.1. The tibial longitudinal residual growth (M±SD)

	Total length of tibia (mm)				The loss of total length of "R" in comparison to final length of "L" in M6 period		The growth in length for D 0 – M 6 period		
	D 0		M 6				Of segment total length for M6 (%)		The loss of length of "R" in comparison to "L" (%)
	«R»	«L»	«R»	«L»	mm	%	«R»	«L»	
Series 1	136.5±39.5	136.7±39.4	152.7±36.7[1]	156.5±37.3[1]	3.8±2.9	2.5±2.1	11.5±5.0	13.6±4.6	17±12.3
Series 2	139.2±9.5	139.2±9.5	172.5±9.8[1]	180.3±8.5[1]	7.8±8.0	4.3±4.3	19.3±3.6	22.8±3.7	14.9±14.0

Note: [1] – statistically significant differences with the initial values of this series.
«R» – right tibia; «L» – left tibia.

Table II.2. Values of proximal medial tibial angle (mMPTA)

		D 0		M 6		M 6 – D 0
		M ± SD (min-max)	P_1	M ± SD (min-max)	P_2	P_3 / P_4
Series 1	Right tibia	91.7°±2.4 (87°-96°)	P^t=0.914	90.8°± 2.1 (88°-94°)	P^t=0.642	P^t=0.306
	Left tibia	90.9°±2.8 (84°-95°)		93.4°±2.3 (90°-99°)		P^t=0.101
Series 2	Right tibia	92.3°±2.1 (90°-95°)	P^t=0.481	91.8 ± 1.9 (90°-95°)	P^t=0.079	P^t=0.675
	Left tibia	91.5±1.9 (89°-94°)		90.0 ± 1.1 (89°-92°)		P^t=0.128

Note: P^1= p-values when compared the right and left side for D0; P^2= p-values when compared the right and left side for M6; P^3= p-values of the right side values for D 0 vs M 6; P^4= p- values of the left side values for D0 vs M6; P^t: p-values for Student's test.

Table II.3. Values of lateral distal tibial angle (mLDTA)

		D 0		M 6		M 6 – D 0
		M ± SD (min-max)	P_1	M ± SD (min-max)	P_2	P_3 / P_4
Series 1	Right tibia	85.2°±3.1 (81°-89°)	P^t=0.563	88.2° ± 5.3 (84°-96°)	P^t=0.023 P^W=0.045	P^t=0.267
	Left tibia	84.2±2.7 (79-87)		81.2° ± 2.8 (76°-84°)		P^t=0.088
Series 2	Right tibia	87.7° ± 2.1 (86°-91°)	P^t=0.718	84.2° ± 6.4 (78°-96°)	P^t=0.691	P^t=0.251
	Left tibia	87.2° ± 2.6 (84°-91°)		83°±2.5 (80°-85°)		$P^{t=}$0.016 P^W=0.026

Note: P^1= p-values when compared the right and left side for D0; P^2= p-values when compared the right and left side for M6; P^3= p-values of the right side values for DS vs M6; P^4= p-values of the left side values for D0 vs M6; P^t: p-values for Student's test; P^W : p-values for non-parametric Wilcoxon test.

Table II.4. Diameter (mm) at the level of middle third in the tibial shaft

	D 0 (AP view)		M 6 (AP view)		D 0 (lateral view)		M 6 (lateral view)	
	right	left	Right	left	right	left	right	left
Series 1	11.3±0.82	11.3±0.82	13.2±0.84[1]	13.2±0.84[1]	10±1.55	10±1.55	11.8±1.72	11.2±1.47
Series 2	12.2±1.17	12.2±1.17	17.2±1.94[1]	14.3±1.21[1 2]	11.2±1.17	11.2±0.75	17.2±1.83[1]	13.3±1.21[2]

Note:

[1] – significant differences D 0 vs M 6 for this series.

[2] – significant differences between right and left sides at M 6.

By the end of the experiment mLDTA values of the experimental (right) segment didn't change statistically significantly among themselves and comparing with the preoperative level in all the series. It can be mentioned that this value had a tendency to increase in the first series for the right limb, and that to some reduction – in the second series. As for the control segment, a reliable decrease in the mLDTA angle was revealed by the end of growth comparing with the preoperative values in the both series (Table II.3).

Thus, in our experiment the transphyseal insertion of elastic nails through the medial malleolus resulted in significant slowing down of the physiological decrease of mLDTA angle (physiological valgus deviation of the ankle) in series II.

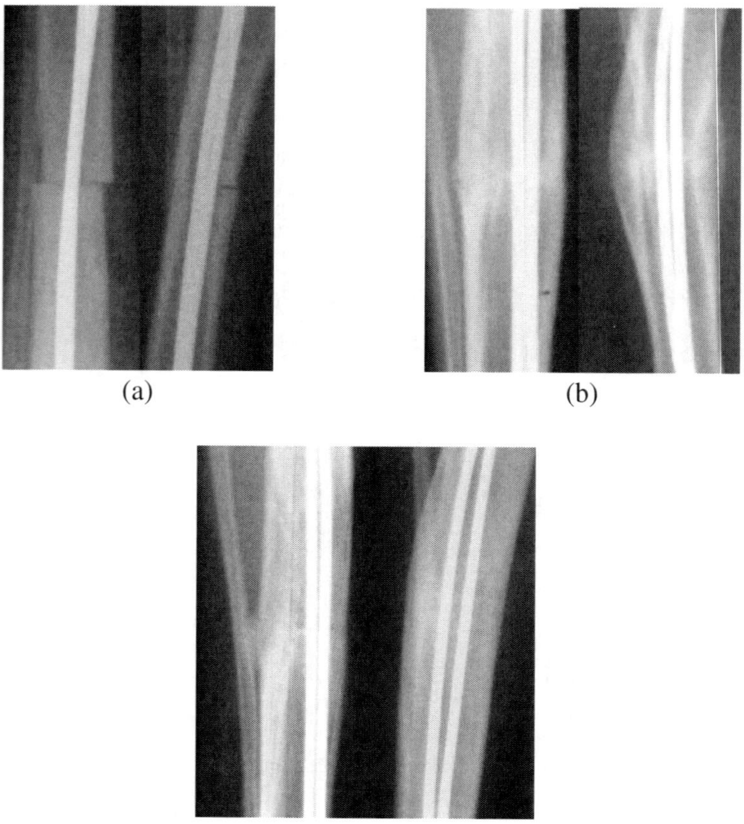

(a) (b) (c)

Figure 11. Bone consolidation (X-rays, AP and lateral views), series II: D 0 (**a**); M 2 (**b**); M 6 (**c**).

The change in the values of tibial outer diameter in the middle third occurred upwards in the right and left limbs of all the animals. Significant difference between D 0 and M 6 were observed in series I and II. According to Table II.4 data, the increase of shaft diameter was the same for operated and intact limb in series I. As we believe, it points out to an immaterial impact of intramedullary elastic nails on the functional activity of both endosteal lining and periosteum.

The X-ray signs of bone consolidation (disappearance of fracture line, continuity of cortical plates) in series II were observed in all the cases by the end of the second month of the experiment (Figure 11). Secondary displacement of fragments was observed in one animal only being characterized by 7° antecurvation deformity. A significant increase of bone diameter in the animals of this series was observed by the end of the experiment, if we compare both with the initial data and between the control and experimental limbs (Table II.4). It is interesting that the most marked periosteal reaction and, consequently, cortical plate thickening occurred on the posterior surface of tibia. It is obvious that osteotomy is a prerequisite for periosteal reaction development under the conditions of the study.

DISCUSSION

Reconstructive orthopaedic interventions in the limbs for the systemic diseases accompanied by bone tissue fragility are intended to prevent deformities or to correct them. A positive effect of such surgeries on patients' functional condition and increase of their motor activity is indisputable [9,10,14-16]. Boutaud and Laville [11] consider that using of intramedullary sliding transphyseal elastic nailing for these purposes is preferable than telescopic rods: no problems with moving elastic nails apart, less total number of complications than with other systems, less incidence of implant migration. Many colleagues performing reconstructive surgeries in children with osteogenesis imperfecta note the common difficulties and/or disadvantages of telescopic systems: need to replace them as far as the child grows, migration of rods or their parts (e.g., threaded ones) when "anchoring" it to the bone (10.5% - 23.7%), telescopic rod deformation (up to 18.8%), the rod fails to elongate (up to 2.1%), the rod's damage (up to 6.9%) [8,17-21]. Thus, the problem of improving telescopic transphyseal systems remains relevant. Moreover, none of clinical studies assesses quantitatively the effect of transphyseally inserted elements on the limb's longitudinal growth, formation of the reinforced segments' epiphyses, or development of angular deformity.

The results of experimental studies on the effect of partial damage of the growth plates varied, but few in number. A negative effect of reaming of the transphyseal canal on the growth function of cartilage was observed in experimental studiesof the proximal tibial physis when they simulated the anterior ligament reconstruction of the tibia. Thus, Chudik [22] and Ono [23] performing the anterior cruciate ligament reconstruction in puppies and rabbits found a statistically significant shortening of the operated segment by the end of natural growth. On the other hand, the straight transphyseally inserted wires of 1.3-2 mm in diameter left in place for less than 12 weeks didn't cause growth dysfunction and consequently shortening in rabbits [24-28]. Epiphyseodesis with this size of wires was observed within the period of 12-24 weeks of transphyseal placement of implants [25,27]. Epiphysiodesis was observed if the wires' diameter exceeded 3.2-3.5 mm [27,28]. Finally, Mäkelä [28] found that injury of over 7% of the growth plate area led to an irreversible epiphysiodesis and segment shortening. On the other hand, the use of biodegradable transphyseal thin rods in rats doesn't lead to epiphysiodesis [29].

In clinical practice, especially in traumatology, the authors' opinion about the effect of transphyseal wire insertion on the growth cartilage function varies. For example, Horn J. et al. describe partial epiphysiodesis and development of angulation during fracture treatment in children [30]. In turn, Yung and Langenhan do not observe the effect of transphyseally inserted Kirschner wires on further growth of the operated limb [31,32].

In our study the injury of physis area was below 6% when the implants remained in place for 25 weeks, and they didn't cause irreversible epiphysiodesis and formation of statistically significant segment shortening. However, the mean length loss was 3.8 mm in series I, and 7.8 mm – in series II. Transphyseal reinforcement with osteotomy (series II) caused a greater shortening of the operated segment. The loss of residual growth of the operated segment was from 14% to 18%. Thus, the growth retardation was found in all the series of our study.

In our study, intramedullary sliding transphyseal nailing influenced the formation of the angle of inclination of the distal tibial articular surface. Eccentric placement of intramedullary nails through the medial malleolus led either to the ankle varus deviation (in series I) with a significant difference between the control limb and experimental one by the end of growth, or, as in series II, to significant inhibition of physiological valgus deviation (mLDTA decrease).

Central transphyseal placement of the nails didn't cause significant angular deviation in any series of the study. Studies of other authors confirm the fact of angular deviation in case of eccentric injury of the growth plate. In 1994 Guzzanti found two cases of knee valgus development because of lateral location of transphyseal canal and tendon insertion into it in their experimental series of the anterior cruciate ligament plasty in 21 rabbits [33]. Seil did not observe angular deviation during residual growth of the segment following a centrally located channel in 18 lambs [34]. The above mentioned studies and our own data confirm the position of Ford [35], that the central injury of the growth plate doesn't cause angular deformities, but can contribute to segment shortening formation, and peripheral epiphyseodesis leads to angular deformity development.

It is important to mention that long presence of the implant is essential for growth function modification in addition to topography and extent of growth plate injury. There are several studies, which demonstrated that acute forming of the transphyseal canel without wire or tendon placement doesn't lead to epiphyseodesis, as well as doesn't cause any disorders of longitudinal bone growth [36,37]. While formation of a narrow epiphyseodesis zone surrounding the permanently present implant is an irreversible cause of growth inhibition in this part of physis [38,39]. At the same time, just a relatively small size of epiphysiodesis (below 7%) allows spontaneous desepiphysiodesis in the process of active growth [28]. We think that repeated epiphysiodeses and spontaneous desepiphysiodeses explain local inhibition of physis function resulting in growth retardation, but not in arrest of growth immediately after surgery.

Both endosteal and periosteal reactions observed during experimental fracture treatment using intramedullary elastic nails are described in some studies [13,40]. The reasons are those referred to the mechanical irritation of medullary canal inner surface on one hand, and those referred to the redistribution of cortical plate blood flow to peripheral structures on the other hand. The endosteal and periosteal reactions in our experimental series were observed as well. However, there was no periosteal reaction in the first series, and the marked endosteal osteogenesis at the level of the contact with nail ends contributed to cortical plate thickening and bone envelope formation around the intramedullary nails. The periosteal reaction was noted in the second series, where bone integrity damage and periosteum detachment were produced. Thus, we believe that itwas just a direct mechanical impact that initiated endosteal and periosteal osteogenesis in our study.

It should be mentioned, that we didn't observe disorders of wires moving apart during growth in the medullary canal in the first series, where the segment preventive reinforcement was imitated. These data confirmed the results reported by Boutard and Laville [11], and they demonstrated the advantages of intramedullary sliding elastic nailing over the telescopic rods from this point of view. However, locking of the elastic nail sliding was observed in three cases when bone fracture was simulated (series II). In our opinion, blocking of the nails with endosteal callus at the level of osteotomy may be an obstacle to moving the rods apart.

The intramedullary elastic osteosynthesis for treatment of shaft fractures in children, including pathological ones, is the most common and reliable surgical method used by pediatric orthopedists of many countries [13,41]. It is quite natural that consolidation of bone fragments took place in all the cases and within usual delay in series II of our study.

The encouraging results of using bisphosphonates [22,26,39] and/or implants with bioactive coating [42] in patients with osteogenesis imperfecta encourages us to hope that combination of therapeutic and surgical methods of treatment will contribute to improve the outcomes in terms of both anatomical (longitudinal growth of segments and prevention of deformities) and functional results of treatment.

Conclusion

This experimental study has demonstrated that transphyseal elastic osteosynthesis influences on the segment longitudinal growth. The least length loss was observed in the intramedullary sliding transphyseal nailing simulating preventive osteosynthesis.

The eccentric insertion of transphyseal nails causes angular deformity development or slows down the physiological orientation of articular surface. Thus, transphyseal telescopic systems should provide positioning of implant elements in the center of growth plates only.

Endosteal and periosteal reactions to intramedullary implant insertion lead to increase of cortical plate thickness and bone diameter, that may be benificial in case of combined treatment of osteogenesis imperfecta by pharmacological and surgical methods.

REFERENCES

[1] Sofield, H. A. & Millar, E. A. (1959). Fragmentation, realignment, and intramedullary rod fixation of deformities of the long bones in children. *J Bone Joint Surg Am.*, *41*, 1371–1391.

[2] Bailey, R. W. & Cole, W. G. (1993). Early surgical management of severe forms of osteogenesis imperfecta. *Am J Med Genet.*, *45*. 270-274.

[3] Bailey, R. W. & Dubow, H. I. (1963). Studies of longitudinal bone growth resulting in an extensible nail. *Surg Forum.*, *14*, 455-458.43. Popkov A., Popkov D. (2012). Bioactif Implants in Traumatology and Orthopaedics [in russian]. Irkutsk., Russia: *NSRS SO RAMN.*, 438p.

[4] Ryöppy, S., Alberty, A. & Kaitila, I. (1987). Early semiclosed intramedullary stabilization in osteogenesis imperfecta. *J Pediatr Orthop.*, *7*(2), 139-144.

[5] Tiley, F. & Albright, J. A. (1973). Osteogenesis imperfecta: treatment by multiple osteotomy and intramedullary rod insertion. Report on thirteen patients. *J Bone Joint Surg Am.*, *55*(4), 701-713.

[6] Williams, P. F. (1965). Fragmentation and rodding in Osteogenesis Imperfecta. *J Bone Joint Surg Br.*, *47*, 23-31.

[7] Metaizeau, J. P. (1987). Sliding centro-medullary nailing. Application to the treatment of severe forms of osteogenesis imperfecta. *Chir Pediatr.*, *28*, 240-243.

[8] El-Adl, G., Khalil, M. A., Enan, A., Mostafa, M. F.,& El-Lakkany, M. R. (2009). Telescoping versus non-telescoping rods in the treatment of osteogenesis imperfecta. *Acta Orthop Belg.*, *75*(2), 200-208.

[9] Ruck, J., Dahan-Oliel, N., Montpetit, K., Rauch, F. & Fassier, F. (2011). Fassier-Duval femoral rodding in children with osteogenesis imperfecta receiving bisphosphonates: functional outcomes at one year. *J Child Orthop.*, *5*(3), 217-224.

[10] Wirth, T. (2012). Osteogenesis imperfecta. *Orthop.*, *41*(9), 773-782.

[11] Boutaud, B. & Laville, J. M. (2004). L'embrochage centromédullaire coulissant dans l'ostéogenèse imparfaite. *Rev Chir Orthop.*, *90*, 304-311.

[12] Salter, R. B. & Harris, W. R. (1963). Injuries involving the epiphyseal plate. *J Bone Jt Surg.*, *45*(3), 587-622.

[13] Lascombes, P. (2010). Flexible intramedullary nailing. *Springer-Verlag Berlin Heidelberg.*

[14] Esposito, P. & Plotkin, H. (2008). Surgical treatment of osteogenesis imperfecta: current concepts. *Curr Opin Pediatr.*, *20*, 52–57.

[15] Khoshhal, K. I. & Ellis, R. D. (2001). Functional outcome of Sofield procedure in the upper limb in osteogenesis imperfecta. *J Pediatr Orthop.*, *21*(2), 236-237.

[16] Porat, S., Heller, E., Seidman, D. S. & Meyer S. (1991). Functional results of operation in osteogenesis imperfecta: elongating and nonelongating rods. *J Pediatr Orthop.*, *11*, 200–203.

[17] Gamble, J. G., Strudwick, W. J., Rinsky, L. A. & Bleck, E. E. (1988). Complications of intramedullary rods in osteogenesis imperfecta: Bailey-Dubow rods versus nonelongating rods. *J Pediatr Orthop.*, *8*, 645-649.

[18] Glorieux, F. H. (2007). Treatment of osteogenesis imperfecta: who., why., what? *Horm Res.*, *68*, Suppl 5, 8-11.

[19] Glorieux, F. H. (2008). Osteogenesis imperfecta. *Best Pract Res Clin Rheumatol.*, *22*, 85–100.

[20] Monti, E., Mottes, M., Fraschini, P., Brunelli, PC., Forlino, A., Venturi, G., Doro, F., Perlini, S., Cavarzere, P. & Antoniazzi. (2010). Current and emerging treatments for the management of osteogenesis imperfecta. *Ther Clin Risk Manag.*, *6*, 367–381.

[21] Zionts, L. E., Ebramzadeh, E. & Stoot, N. S. (1998). Complications in the use of the Bailey-Dubow extensible wire. *Clin Orthop. 18*, 102-109.

[22] Chudik, S., Beasley, L., Potter, H., Wickiewicz, T., Warren, R. & Rodeo, S. (2007). The influence of femoral technique for graft placement on anterior cruciate ligament reconstruction using a skeletally immature canine model with a rapidly growing physis. *Arthrosc J Arthrosc Relat Surg Off Publ Arthrosc Assoc North Am Int Arthrosc Assoc.*, *23*(12), 1309-1319.

[23] Ono, T., Wada, Y., Takahashi, K., Tsuchida, T., Minamide, M. & Moriya, H. (1998). Tibial deformities and failures of anterior cruciate ligament reconstruction in immature rabbits. *J Orthop Sci Off J Jpn Orthop Assoc.*, *3*(3), 150-155.

[24] Boelitz, R., Dallek, M., Meenen, N. M. & Jungbluth, K. H. (1994). Reaction of the epiphyseal groove to groove-crossing bore-wire osteosynthesis. Results of a histomorphologic small animal study. *Unfallchirurgie.*, *20*(3), 131-137.

[25] Cady, R. B., Siegel, J. A., Mathien, G., Spadaro, J. A. & Chase, S. E. (1999). Physeal response to absorbable polydioxanone bone pins in growing rabbits. *J Biomed Mater Res.*, *48*(3), 211-215.

[26] Hajdu, S., Schwendenwein, E., Kaltenecker, G., László, I., Lang, S., Vécsei, V. & Sarahrudi, K. (2011). The effect of drilling and screw fixation of the growth plate - an experimental study in rabbits. *J Orthop Res.*, *29*(12), 1834-1839.

[27] Kameyama, M. (1993). An experimental study on injuries to the growth plate - effects on the growth of long bones following placement of smooth pins across the growth plate of immature rabbits. *Nihon Seikeigeka Gakkai Zasshi.*, *67*(7), 662-676.

[28] Mäkelä, E. A., Vainionpää, S., Vihtonen, K., Mero, M. & Rokkanen, P. (1988). The effect of trauma to the lower femoral epiphyseal plate. An experimental study in rabbits. *J Bone Joint Surg Br.*, *70*(2), 187-191.

[29] Fischerauer, S., Kraus, T., Wu, X., Tandl, S., Sorantin, E., Hanzi, A. C., Loffler, J. F., Uggowitzer, P. J. & Weinberg, A. M. (2013). In vivo degradation performance of micro-arc-oxidized implants: a micro-CT study in rats. *Acta Biomater*, 2013., *9*(2), 5411-5420.

[30] Horn, J., Kristiansen, L. P. & Steen, H. (2008). Partial physeal arrest after temporary transphyseal pinning. A case report. *Acta Orthop.*, *79*(6), 867-869.

[31] Langenhan, R., Baumann, M., Hohendorff, B., Probst, A. & Trobisch, P. (2013). Arthroscopically assisted reduction and internal fixation of a femoral anterior cruciate ligament osteochondral avulsion fracture in a 14-year-old girl via transphyseal inside-out technique. *Strategies Trauma Limb Reconstr.*, *8*(3), 193–197.

[32] Yung, P. S., Lam, C. Y., Ng, B. K., Lam, T. P. & Cheng, J. C. (2004). Percutaneous transphyseal intramedullary Kirschner wire pinning: a safe and effective procedure for treatment of displaced diaphyseal forearm fracture in children. *J Pediatr Orthop.*, *24*(1), 7-12.

[33] Guzzanti, V., Falciglia, F., Gigante, A. & Fabbriciani, C. (1994). The effect of intra-articular ACL reconstruction on the growth plates of rabbits. *J Bone Joint Surg Br.*, *76*(6), 960-963.

[34] Seil, R., Pape, D. & Kohn, D. (2008). The risk of growth changes during transphyseal drilling in sheep with open physes. *Arthrosc J Arthrosc Relat Surg Off Publ Arthrosc Assoc North Am Int Arthrosc Assoc.*, *24*(7), 824-833.

[35] Ford, L. T. & Key, J. A. (1956). A study of experimental trauma to the distal femoral epiphysis in rabbits. *J Bone Joint Surg Am. 38*-A(1), 84-92.

[36] Campbell, C. J., Grisolia, A. & Zanconato, G. (1959). The effects produced in the cartilaginous epiphyseal plate of immature dogs by experimental surgical traumata. *J Bone Joint Surg Am.*, 41-A, 1221-1242.

[37] Nordentoft, E. L. (1969). Experimental epiphyseal injuries. Grading of traumas and attempts at treating traumatic epiphyseal arrest in animals. *Acta Orthop Scand.*, *40*(2), 176-192.

[38] Babu, L. V., Evans, O., Sankar, A., Davies, A. G., Jones, S. & Fernandes, J. A. (2014). Epiphysiodesis for limb length discrepancy: a comparison of two methods. *Strategies Trauma Limb Reconstr.*, *9*(1), 1–3.

[39] Stevens, P. M. (2006). Guided growth: 1933 to the present. *Strategies Trauma Limb Reconstr.*, *1*(1), 29–35.

[40] Téot, L. (1987). L'enclouage centromédullaire élastique stable chez l'enfant. Cah Enseign SOFCOT. Elsevier Masson. Paris. 71-90.

[41] Knorr, P., Schmittenbecher, P. P. & Dietz, H. G. (1996). Treatment of pathological fractures of long tubular bones in childhood using elastic stable intramedullary nailing. *Unfallchirurg.*, *99*(6), 410-414.

[42] el-Sobky, M. A., Hanna, A. A., Basha, N. E., Tarraf, Y. N. & Said, M. H. (2006). Surgery versus surgery plus pamidronate in the management of osteogenesis imperfecta patients: a comparative study. *J Pediatr Orthop, B. 15*(3), 222-228.

In: Combined Stimulating Methods …
Editor: Dmitry Popkov
ISBN: 978-1-63483-028-7

Chapter III

LENGTHENING AND DEFORMITY CORRECTION OF LOWER AND UPPER LIMBS

Pierre Lascombes, PhD, MD[1], Arnold Popkov, PhD, MD.[2], Pierre Journeau, PhD, MD[3], and Dmitry Popkov, PhD, MD[2*]

[1]Pediatric Orthopedic Surgery Dept, Geneva University Hospitals, Children's Hospital, Geneva, Switzerland

[2]Scientific and Clinical Laboratory for Deformity Correction and Limb Lengthening. Federal Russian State-Financed Ilizarov Scientific Center for Restorative Traumatology and Orthopaedics, Kurgan, Russia

[3]Pediatric Orthopedic Surgery Dept, Nancy University Hospital Center, Children's Hospital, Vandoeuvre, France

ABSTRACT

Background. The aim of this study is to evaluate the influence of the external fixation associated with intramedullary nailing on the healing index in limb lengthening.

Material and Methods. This study was based on a series of patients with lower and upper limb length discrepancy of different etiologies. We

* Corresponding author: Ilizarov Scientific Center for Restorative Traumatology and Orthopaedics, 6, M.-Ulyanova Street, 640014 Kurgan, Russia; dpopkov@mail.ru,

evaluated results of treatment in patients undergoing limb lengthening with the combination of an external circular fixator and intramedullary nailing (154 cases). The Ilizarov frame (133 cases) or Taylor Spatial Frame (21 cases) were used in combination with flexible intramedullary nailing.

Results. In all the groups of patients we observed a significant reduction of the Healing Index – inferior to 30 days/cm. There were 117 complications but only 10 of them influenced on results of treatment. Finally, results are distributed according to categories: I category – 114 cases (74%), IIa – 27 cases (17.5%), IIb – 3 cases (1.9%), IIIa – 9 cases (5.7%), IVa – 1 case (0.9%).

Conclusion. Flexible intramedullary nailing provides multiple advantages to a method of limb lengthening. Flexible Intramedullary Nailing, when correctly applied, respects the bone biological features which are essential for successful limb lengthening. The major effect of application of the combination of external circular fixation with FIN is significant decrease of external osteosynthesis duration.

Keywords: Bone lengthening, Ilizarov method, flexible intramedullary nailing, Taylor spatial frame

INTRODUCTION

Gradual lengthening is the most reliable method in treatment of length discrepancy of upper and lower limb segments. Since the 80-s of the 20th century various changes of operative technique have been introduced aiming to improve the anatomic and functional results and to reduce duration of external fixation: lengthening in automatic mode, stimulation by acute compression of the regenerate, bifocal and polysegmental lengthening [1-3].

Actually, there are two possibilities to combine external fixation and intramedullary nailing in bone lengthening. The first one is presented by an association of external fixator and rigid intramedullary nail of 10 mm and more in diameter [4-6]. The second type of combined technique unites the external fixation and *flexible* intramedullary nailing [3, 7-9].

The experimental study described in the first chapters of this book proved that use of flexible intramedullary nails provides a favourable effect on formation of distraction regenerate. Encouraged by the experimental series, a clinical study was launched, in 2001 in an adolescent affected with a congenital shortening of a lower limb. Currently our technique takes a reliable and important place in the therapeutic arsenal of pediatric orthopedics.

The aim of this study is to demonstrate how the flexible intramedullary nailing influences the outcome in lengthening of upper and lower limbs.

MATERIAL AND METHODS

We have studied results of 154 limb lengthenings in patients of the age between 3 to 22 years old (the mean age at the beginning of lengthening was 11.2±0.17). Lengthening was performed in 79 cases in girls and in 75– in boys.

Lengthening was performed with the Ilizarov fixator (121 cases) or Taylor Space Frame (TSF®) (33) during the period 2001 - 2008 in two clinics: in the Ilizarov Scientific Center for Restorative Traumatology and Orthopaedics (Kurgan, Russia) and in the Children's Hospital of Nancy University Hospital Center (Nancy, France). Surgery was performed by the authors of this study during the years 2001 - 2010.

An inclusion criterion was upper or lower limb lengthening performed with the combined technique if results could be assessed in 12 months minimum after frame removal.

Table III.1. Variants of distraction osteosynthesis in lower limb lengthening

Segment	Type of distraction osteosynthesis	Congenital		Acquired		Faralytic		Ollier disease		Neurofibromatosis, fibrous dysplasia	
		Nb	Mean age	Nb	Mean age	Nb	Age	Nb	Mean age	Nb	Age
Femur	Monofocal+ FIN	19	12.5± 0.98	9	13.7± 0.9	1	16	4	12.5± 1.9	1	8
	Biforal+FIN	7	11.2± 1.7	5	12.2± 0.6						
Tibia	Monofocal+ FIN	22	11.3± 1.17	6	9± 1.5	1	15	1	11		
	Biforal+FIN	7	11.7± 2.1	2	15± 1.0						
Femur+ Tibia	Polysegmental +FIN	13	13.2± 0.8	6	11.7± 1.4			2	16.5± 3.2	1	14
Total		68		28		2		7		2	

Table III.2. Variants of distraction osteosynthesis in upper limb lengthening

Segment	Type of distraction osteosynthesis	Congenital		Acquired		Paralytic		Exostotic disease	
		Nb	Mean age	Nb	Mean age	Nb	Mean age	Nb	Mean age
Humerus	Monofocal+FIN	3	10± 6.0	3	9.7± 2.19	2	11.5± 3.5		
	Bifocal+FIN			13	13± 0.59	1	16		
Forearm	Monofocal+FIN	18	9.9± 1.04	3	13± 0.58	1	16	2	6.5±0.5
Humerus+Forearm	Polysegmental+FIN	1	7						
Total		22		19		4		2	

The distribution of cases according to the aetiology, type of distraction osteosynthesis, mean age at the beginning of lengthening is presented in Tables III.1 and III.2.

It is worth of mentioning that in the group of acquired discrepancy the limb length inequality developed as a result of post-traumatic epiphysiolysis or the physis damaged by the hematogenous osteomyelitis or osteoarthritis. Sequela of hematogenous osteomyelitis caused the lower limb length discrepancy in 15 cases, premature posttraumatic closure of the growth plate in 13 cases. Among the upper limb length discrepancy, sequela of osteomyelitis was observed in 12 children, consequences of the physis lesion – in 7 cases. For the group of paralytic shortening the reason of length inequality of lower limbs (2 pts) was poliomyelitis, of upper limbs (4 pts) – the obstetrical trauma of a brachial plexus.

Monosegmental monofocal osteosynthesis in combination with FIN of the femur or tibia was done in 64 cases. Monosegmental bifocal distraction osteosynthesis of the femur or tibia was applied in 21 cases. Polysegmental distraction osteosynthesis of the lower limb was applied in 22 patients.

Monosegmental osteosynthesis in combination with FIN of the humerus was done in 8 cases. Bifocal distraction osteosynthesis of the humerus was applied in 14 cases. Monosegmental osteosynthesis of the forearm was used in 24 cases. Polysegmental distraction osteosynthesis of the upper limb was applied in only 1 patient.

Surgical Technique

The first stage of the surgery, a classical procedure, consists of application of the external fixator followed by the osteotomy via a percutaneous incision that preserves the periosteum and intramedullary vascularization [10, 11].

The second stage is application of FIN: through two incisions of 1 to 2 cm in the metaphyseal area two entry holes are made in the bone very oblique to the osteotomy by means of the trocar of 3-4 mm in diameter at a distance of 1.5 to 3 cm from the growth plate. For the femoral lengthening FIN is retrograde, starting from the distal metaphysis, if the lengthening is performed in the lower third of the segment. For the tibia (Figure 12), it is antegrade through the proximal metaphyseal approach. As for the humerus, the approach is distal at the level of the lateral supracondylar area with a retrograde FIN.

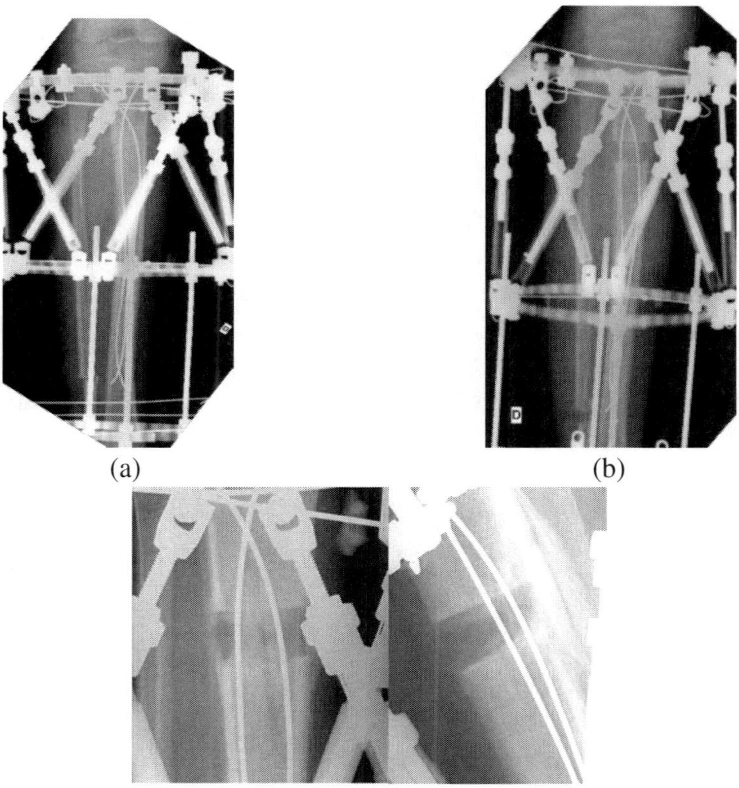

(a) (b) (c)

Figure 12. (Continued).

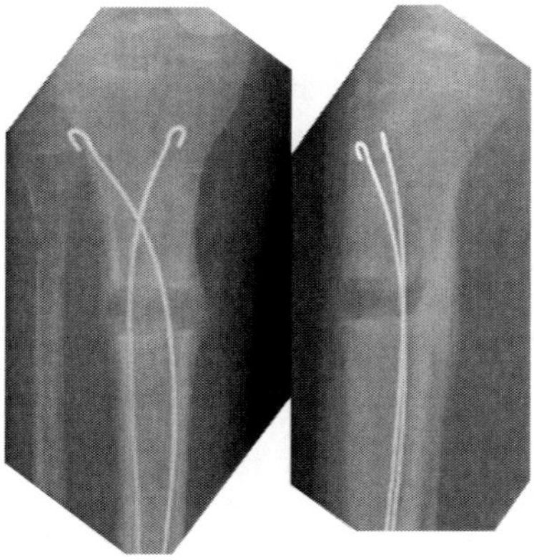

(d)

Figure 12. Surgical technique. Application of two Ilizarov rings, tibial osteoclasia and intramedullary nails. The two curved nails are inserted into the intramedullary canal in anterograde direction. The maximum curves are above the osteoclasia site. Their distal ends are bent (**a**). During the lengthening the nails slide with the proximal fragment (**b**). Note: significant periosteal reaction both at the level of diastasis and at the adjacent bone fragments, regenerate is dense and significant (**c**), after frame removal (**d**).

Two steel or titanium nails of the diameter from 1.5 to 2.5 mm are pre-curved with the ray of curvature about 40 to 60º and their tips of 1.5 to 3 mm are curved at 30 to 40º. The tip of every nail is blunt. The nails must be bent in a way that allows assembling two intersecting arches. The two nails opposed to each other are situated in the same plane creating the same geometric system - elastic and resistant, which is the same for a diaphyseal fracture. An important difference is that the nails have a smaller diameter in comparison to those used for fracture management.

We used intramedullary nails of 20 to 25% of medullary canal diameter in order to avoid its blocking by external fixator wires or half-pins during distraction period.

The two nails must be carefully introduced one by one up to the osteotomy site, then pushed through it until they finally reach the opposite metaphysis. Rotation of the curved blunt tip allows toavoid the half-pins and wires of external fixator, while inserting a nail along medullary canal, straight or deformed. The maximum curve should be placed near the osteotomy site in the diaphyseal part that enables to cross the nails above the osteotomy. In these conditions the lengthening slowly moves the apex of the nail curvature and it is situated at the level of the growing zone of the regenerate by the end of lengthening period (Figure 12).

If a bone segment is straight, the initial curvature of both nails must be identical. In a case of bone deformity, the arch of one nail can be more curved for maintaining a permanent tension that helps the angular correction during the lengthening. Another solution is to reorient both nails, opposing their concavity to the bone deformity.

External tips of intramedullary nails are bent at over 90° to avoid their migration into the medullary canal during the distraction period, and then they are cut as usually 5 to 10 mm from the bone. The skin is sutured.

The bifocal lengthening can also be associated with FIN. In this case a bipolar variant of nailing is more appropriate. Thus, for example, for the tibia, one antegrade nail is inserted through the proximal metaphysis, while the distal retrograde nail is inserted through the distal metaphysis (Figure 13). During the lengthening period the implants slide along one another in the same way as in a technique for the osteogenesis imperfecta. After the frame removal both regenerates remain reinforced at least by one intramedullary nail curved and oriented in a way opposing the natural tendency of the secondary deformity.

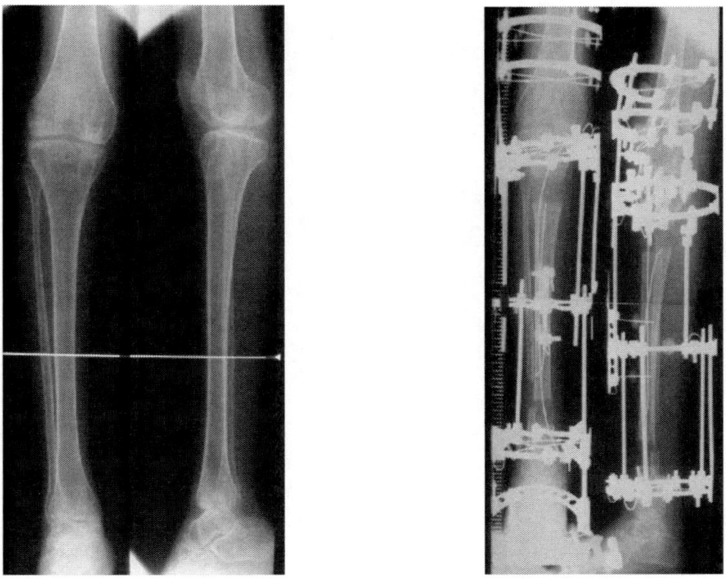

(a) (b)

Figure 13. (Continued),

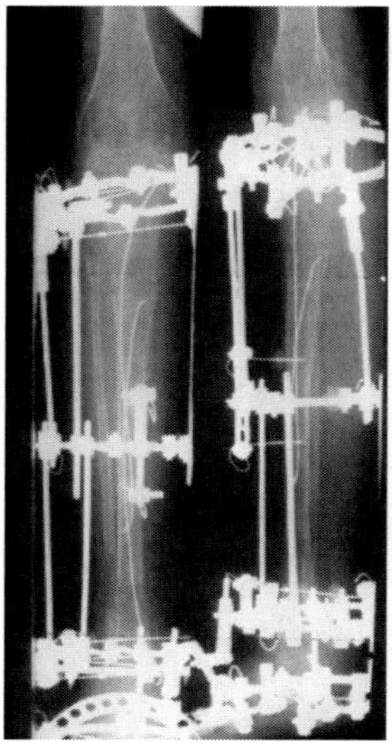

(c)

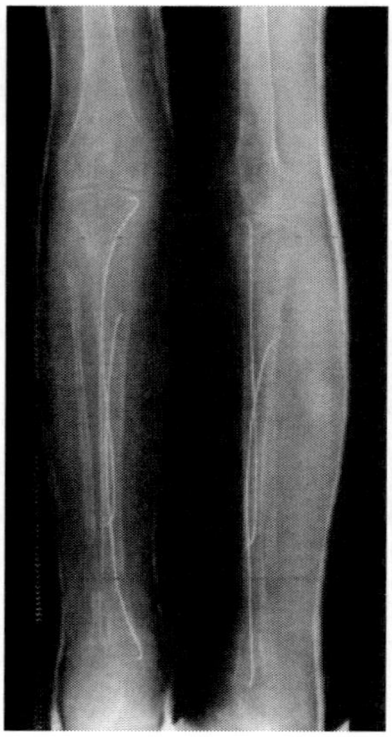

(d)

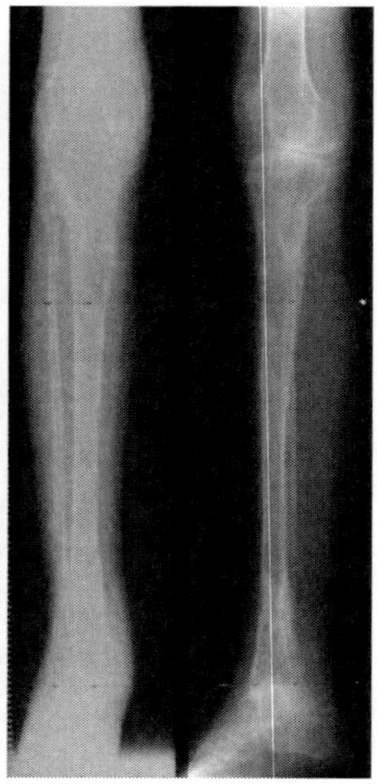

(e)

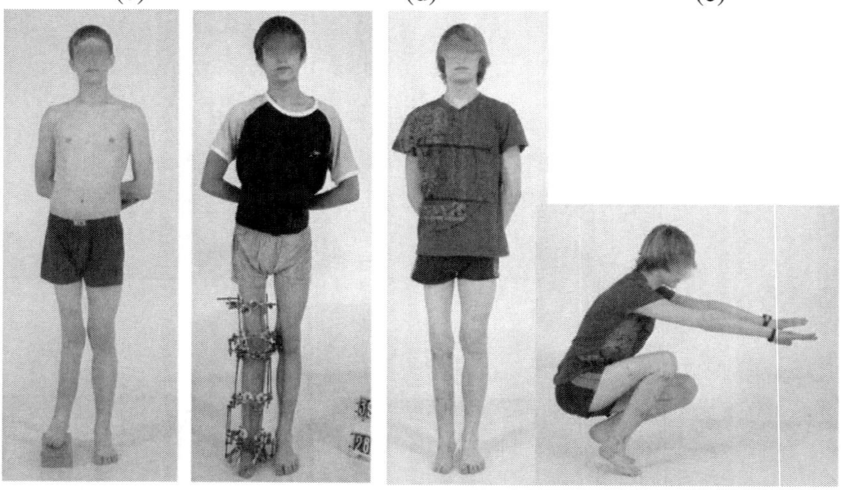

(f)

Figure 13. Bifocal lengthening of tibia: X-rays of the tibia before surgery (**a**), on the 30th day of distraction period (**b**), by the end of fixation period (6 weeks), cortical continuity, disappearance of growth zone of regenerate (**c**), after frame removal, amount of lengthening – 7 cm, HI – 15.6 d/cm (**d**), FIN removal performed in 5 months (**e**), patient before, during and after treatment (**f**).

In a case of forearm lengthening we use a tension assembling with a nail in the radial bone, which concavity is oriented to the ulna, and vice versa in the ulna bone. In all the cases the nailing is retrograde in the radius, inserted through an incision of 1.5-2 cm above the distal physis, avoiding superficial nerves and veins, and it is antegrade in the ulna, inserted through a posterior-lateral approach of the olecranon (Figures 14, 15).

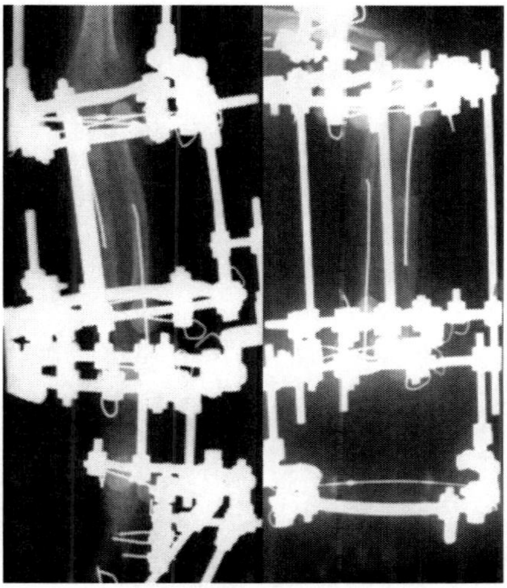

Figure 14. Exemple of forearm lengthening: nailing is retrograde in the radius and antegrade in the ulna.

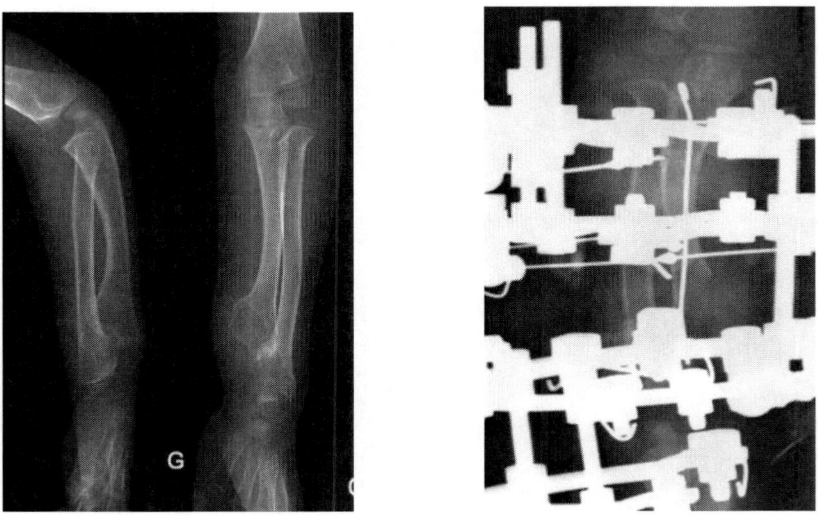

(a) (b)

Figure 15. (Continued).

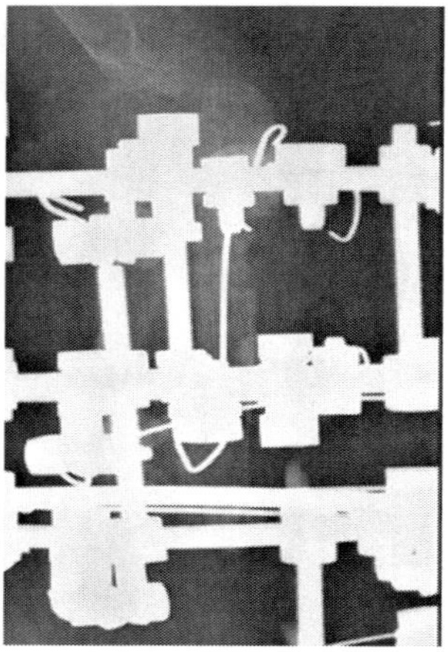

(c)

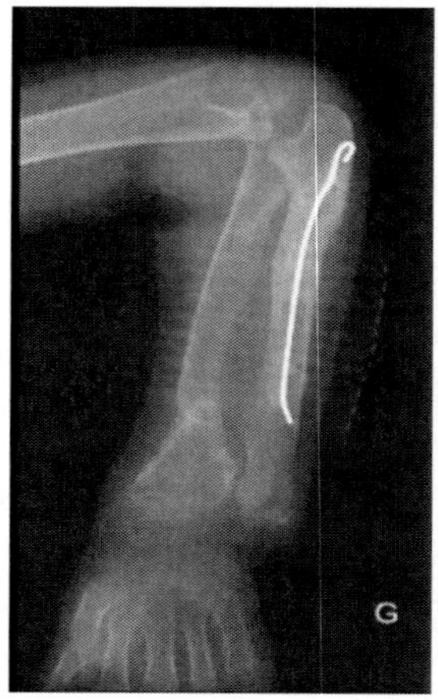

(d)

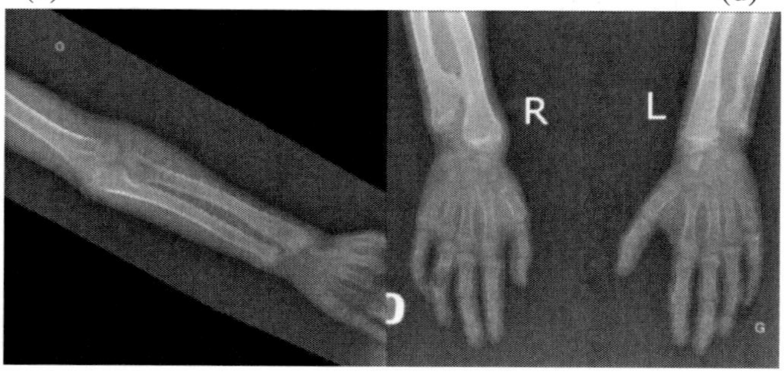

(e)

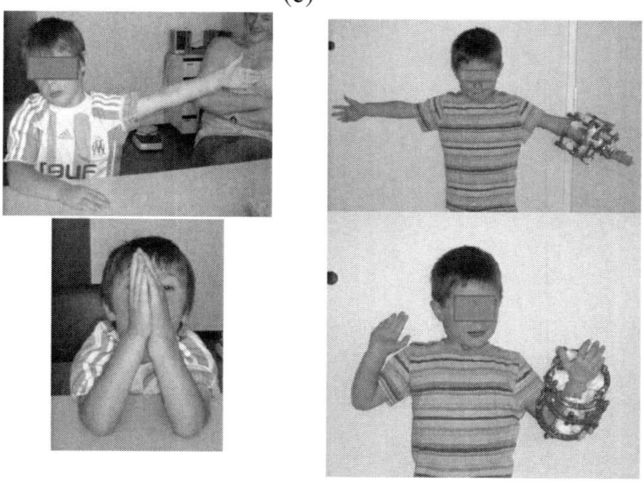

(f)

Figure 15. (Continued).

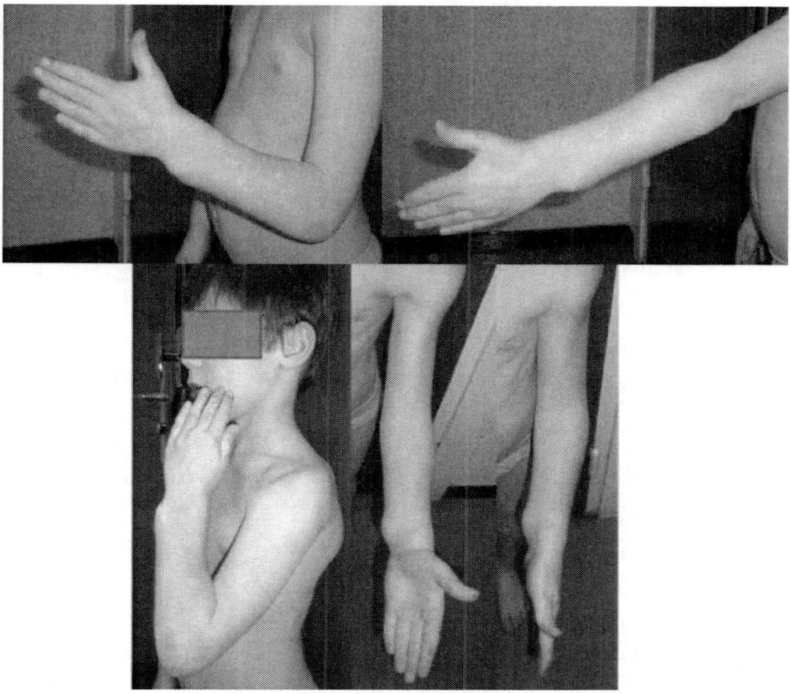

(g)

Figure 15. Forearm lengthening and cubital club hand deformity correction in a boy 6 y.o. with multiple exostoses: X-rays before surgery (**a**), in the beginning of the distraction period, the lengthening of ulna will be performed with intramedullary nailing, the deformity of the distal radius will be without lengthening (**b**), after correction, the first days of fixation period (**c**), after frame removal, gain of lengthening – 4 cm, HI – 22.3 d/cm (**d**), in a year after frame removal et 6 months after FIN removal (**e**), patient before and during treatment (**f**), functional outcome in a year after frame removal (**g**).

A distinction of the external fixator associated with FIN is an ability to attach additional wires or a half-pin after insertion of intramedullary nails. It concerns the frontal wire at a level of the distal femur or proximal tibia or also certain wires of the intermediate ring in the bifocal lengthening. Thus, all the external wires which can interfere the passage of the intramedullary nails in the medullary canal are inserted after FIN.

Lengthening begins on the 4-6th day after the surgery. Limb function is preserved by an early articular mobilization and weight bearing according to usual indications of the lengthening method.

Combined deformities are progressively corrected in all the patients during the lengthening period. With the Ilizarov technique, hinges are positioned according to the center of rotation of angulations CORA [12]. With the TSF®, the correction is progressively obtained simultaneously with lengthening following the instructions of the computerized program [13, 14].

Implants are removed in two steps. The external fixator can be removed at the beginning of bone consolidation according to radiographs and clinical test. A precise date is difficult to determine: when the "growth zone" has disappeared and the radiographic continuity of at least 3 of 4 cortices is observed. Total weight bearing is allowed by the end of six weeks after Ilizarov fixator removal but a semicircular plaster cast is permanently applied for the period of 2 to 4 weeks. The removal of nails is possible in 2 to 8 months after frame removal.

A general classification of results of bone lengthening [15] is applied to evaluate the outcomes.

This classification (Table III.3) is based on the respecting of a triple contract (gain of lengthening, projected treatment duration, and functional outcome):

- grade I: the triple contract is fulfilled, procedures are undertaken under local anesthesia and/or medical treatments are necessary but no intervention under general anesthesia is undertaken;
- grade II: the triple contract is also fulfilled but unscheduled intervention(s) under general anesthesia are necessary. These procedures can take place before the end of the lengthening program (grade II-a) or after the end of this program (grade II-b) without changing the date of external fixator removal;
- grade III: pursuing treatment is necessary beyond the planned period to obtain bone union, but at term, no alteration of function is observed. The HI is therefore lengthened with the external fixator removal or total weight bearing delayed beyond the scheduled time. In grade III-a, the length gain is greater than or equal to 75% of the initial objective, whereas a gain less than 75% is classified as grade III-b. It is possible in grade III-b that bone union takes place within the normal time delay with a HI less than 45 days/cm, but since the scheduled correction has not been obtained, the patient, who desires so, could request a new surgery; this can result in a new therapeutic period;

- grade IV: despite the different treatments, sequelae exist at the final evaluation when the gain is 75% or higher (grade IV-a) or less than 75% (grade IV-b). Whether or not the initial objective of treatment is met, loss of function means worsening of the earlier functional state.

Table III.3. Description of the four-grade classification

Grade	I	II-a	II-b	III-a	III-b	IV-a	IV-b
Surgery with general anesthesia	No	Yes before[a]	Yes after[a]	Possible	Possible	Possible	Possible
Planned length gain obtained	Yes	Yes	Yes	Yes	No	Yes	No
Planned duration respected	Yes	Yes	Yes	No	No	Yes/no	Yes/no
Function respected	Yes	Yes	Yes	Yes	Yes	No	No

[a] Removal of external fixator.

Statistical analysis was performed using the software AtteStat®.

RESULTS

The average amount of lengthening was 5.1±0.2 cm, the relative average amount of lengthening made 20.3% of the initial length of a segment. It is important to assess the relative lengthening for each segment separately, including polysegmental lengthening.

Radiographic evaluation revealed the following features of formation of the distraction regenerate. In our series the regenerate was always dense and significant. In the majority of cases starting from the third week of lengthening the regenerate was well structured and filled the entire gap between the bone fragments. Its “growth zone” was 2 to 5 mm and abundantly filled with bone trabeculae, while the periosteal reaction increased. The diameter of the regenerate exceeded the diameter of bone fragments by 2 to 6 mm because of the periosteal reaction at the level of diastases and adjacent bone fragments as well (Figure 12).

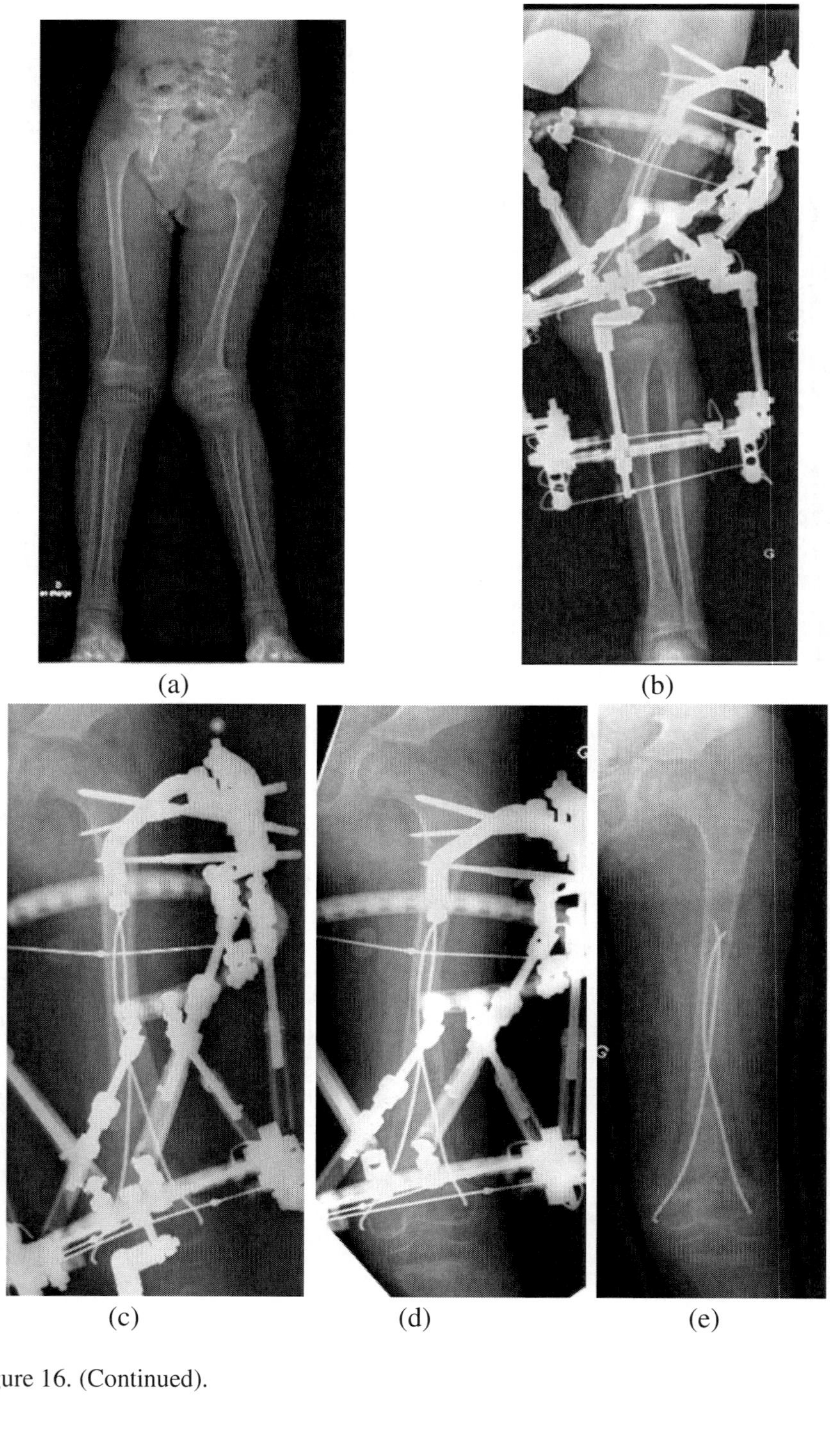

Figure 16. (Continued).

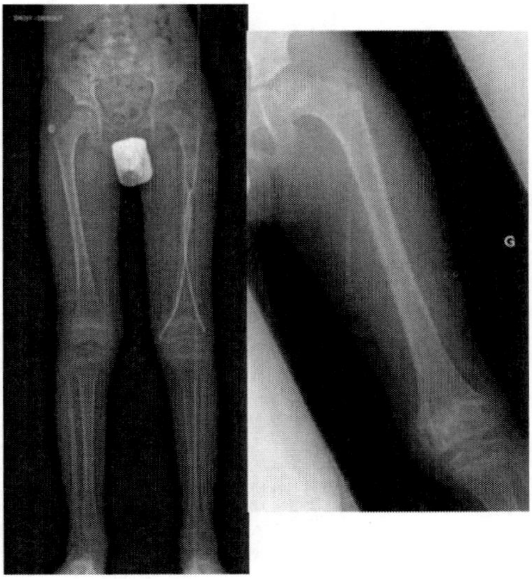

(f)

Figure 16. Femoral monofocal lengthening in a boy presenting posttraumatic lower limb length discrepancy: X-rays before surgery (**a**), on the 7th day of distraction period (**b**), on the 30th day of distraction period (**c**), at the end of distraction period (58 days) (**d**), after frame removal, gain of lengthening – 6 cm, HI – 20.5 d/cm (**e**), in 7 months after frame removal, FIN removal performed (**f**).

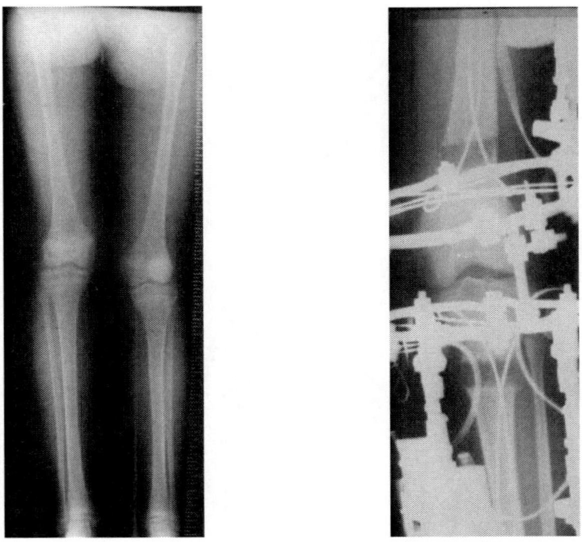

(a) (b)

Figure 17. (Continued).

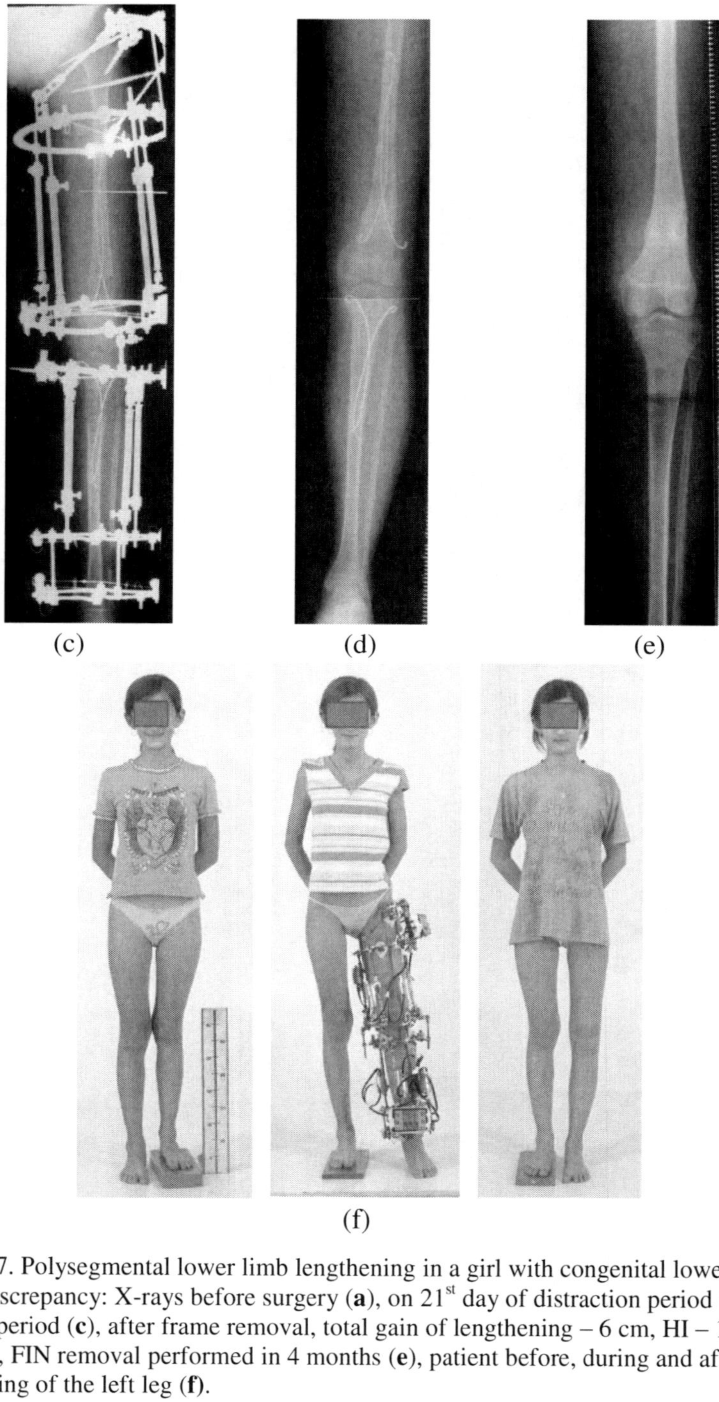

Figure 17. Polysegmental lower limb lengthening in a girl with congenital lower limb length discrepancy: X-rays before surgery (**a**), on 21st day of distraction period (**b**), fixation period (**c**), after frame removal, total gain of lengthening – 6 cm, HI – 15.8 d/cm (**d**), FIN removal performed in 4 months (**e**), patient before, during and after lengthening of the left leg (**f**).

Table III.4. Duration of osteosynthesis, amount of lengthening and healing index in lower limb lengthening

Etiology	Segment	Parameters	Monofocal+FIN	Bifocal+FIN
Congenital	Femur	Osteosynthesis duration; days Lengthening; cm Healing index	91.4± 6.74 4.4± 0.36 21.2± 1.34	117± 7.5 7.0± 0.63 17.6± 2.38
	Tibia	Osteosynthesis duration; days Lengthening; cm Healing index	95.4± 3.65 3.9± 0.31 26.1± 1.74	136.8± 13.95 8.3± 0.802 16.3± 1.97
Acquired	Femur	Osteosynthesis duration; days Lengthening; cm Healing index	74.3± 7.88 4.2± 0.93 18.7± 1.96	98.8± 19.04 8.1± 0.51 12.99± 2.52
	Tibia	Osteosynthesis duration; days Lengthening; cm Healing index	108.7± 7.54 4.5± 0.29 24.3± 1.85	162.5± 39.5 8.5± 0.5 18.9± 3.51
Paralytic	Femur	Osteosynthesis duration; days Lengthening; cm Healing index	145 4.5 29	
	Tibia	Osteosynthesis duration; days Lengthening; cm Healing index	83 25 33.2	
Ollier disease	Femur	Osteosynthesis duration; days Lengthening; cm Healing index	129.1±17.4 5.6±0.62 23.3±2.2	
	Tibia	Osteosynthesis duration; days Lengthening; cm Healing index	112 5 22.4	
Neurofibromatosis	Femur	Osteosynthesis duration; days Lengthening; cm Healing index	96 4.5 21.3	

Tables III.4, III.5 и III.6 present the gain of lengthening and healing index in groups of patients differed by type of external osteosynthesis and etiology of limb length discrepancy (Figures 16 and 17). It is important to note that in all the groups the HI was inferior to 30 days/cm. We can take it as reference data to compare our results with the HI published by other colleagues in "Discussion". Only in one case the HI was 33.2 days/cm in 16 y.o. patient presented paralytic lower limb length discrepancy: monofocal tibial lengthening was performed in sequelae of poliomyelitis.

Table III.5. Duration of osteosynthesis, amount of lengthening and healing index in upper limb lengthening

Etiology	Segment	Parameters	Monofocal+FIN	Bifocal+FIN
Congenital	Humerus	Osteosynthesis duration; days Lengthening; cm Healing index	90.5± 11.5 5± 1.0 19.4± 6.15	
	Forearm	Osteosynthesis duration; days Lengthening; cm Healing index	121.6± 8.79 5.96± 0.36 21.3± 1.53	
Acquired	Humerus	Osteosynthesis duration; days Lengthening; cm Healing index	88.3± 17.95 5.7± 0.88 15.8± 2.31	103.8± 6.9 9.1± 0.59 11.97± 1.29
	Forearm	Osteosynthesis duration; days Lengthening; cm Healing index	85.3± 12.99 3.8± 1.36 26.03± 6.23	
Paralytic	Humerus	Osteosynthesis duration; days Lengthening; cm Healing index	81.5± 2.5 5± 0.0 16.3± 0.5	109 6 18.2
	Forearm	Osteosynthesis duration; days Lengthening; cm Healing index	88 3 29.3	
Hereditary Multiple Exostoses	Forearm	Osteosynthesis duration; days Lengthening; cm Healing index	114.7±7.9 4.1±1.5 27.9±4,3	

Table III.6. Duration of osteosynthesis, amount of lengthening and healing index in polysegmental limb lengthening

Etiology	Limb	Parameters	Fixator+FIN
Congenital	Upper	Osteosynthesis duration; days Lengthening; cm Healing index	112 5.5 20.4
	Lower	Osteosynthesis duration; days Lengthening; cm Healing index	125± 8.7 7.7± 0.6 16.5± 1.24
Acquired	Lower	Osteosynthesis duration; days Lengthening; cm Healing index	115.3± 8.72 6.8± 0.17 16.9± 1.28
Ollier disease	Lower	Osteosynthesis duration; days Lengthening; cm Healing index	138.2±14.8 12.5±0.5 11.6±0.7
Fibrous dysplasia	Lower	Osteosynthesis duration; days Lengthening; cm Healing index	98 5 19.6

Complications were noted in 103 patients (66.9% of cases). The table III.7 presents all the complications observed in our series as well as the treatment applied.

Table III.7. List of complications according to severity grade

Complications	Treatment	Number
Grade I: gain, HI, and function fulfilled - intervention without GA		77
Local infection with pins or wires	Local care ± antibiotic therapy	55
Paresthesia, temporary paralysis	Surveillance, removal of wire in contact, no GA	9
Threat of early bone union	Acceleration of elongation speed	6
Delay in appearance of bone regenerate	Slowing down of elongation speed	2
Migration of FIN	Percutaneous nail pushing, no GA	5
Grade II-a: gain, HI, and function fulfilled - intervention with GA before end of lengthening program		27
Local infection with pins or wires	Pin or wire removal and replacement	7
Migration of FIN nails	Cutting, nail pushing or early removal of FIN nails	7

Table III.7. (Continued)

Complications	Treatment	Number
Problems with ExFix: deviation of assemble, cutaneous contact, instability	Revision of ExFix with GA	4
Breakage of ExFix material, screws	Material removal with GA	5
Early union of regenerate	New osteotomy	3
Infection of osteotomy hematoma	Surgical cleansing and antibiotic therapy	1
Grade II-b: gain, HI, and function fulfilled - intervention with GA after the end of the lengthening program		3
Migration of FIN nails	Early removal of FIN nails	3
Grade III-a: gain and function fulfilled, HI > 45 days/cm		9
Joint stiffness	Mobilization with GA, tendon elongation	6
Fracture and deformity after EF removal	Immobilization cast, epiphysiodesis or osteosynthesis	3
Grade III-b: function fulfilled, gain not obtained, HI > 45days/cm		0
Grade IV-a: function not fulfilled (sequelae), gain obtained		1
Posterior knee subluxation	Secondary progressive correction with EF	1
Grade IV-b: function not fulfilled (sequelae), gain not obtained		0

It should be noted that complications were of I, II-a or II-b categories in 107 cases, meaning the final results of treatment were not compromised and the planned therapeutic objectives were achieved without any sequelae.

We want to emphasize, there were no pathologic fractures after frame removal in patients presenting bone diseases with fragility (Ollier disease, fibrous dysplasia) (Figure 18).

In the majority of cases (143 pts) the intramedullary nails were removed in 3-8 months after removal of the external fixator.

Prior to analysis of treatment results according to the principles of Lascombes classification [15], it is important to mention that 14 patients developed two complications. In such situation a more severe complication has been taken into consideration in assessment of the final result (Figure 19).

Thus, the results were categorized: I – 114 cases (74%), II-a – 27 cases (17.5%), IIb – 3 cases (1.9%), III-a – 9 cases (5.7%), IV-a – 1 case (0.9%).

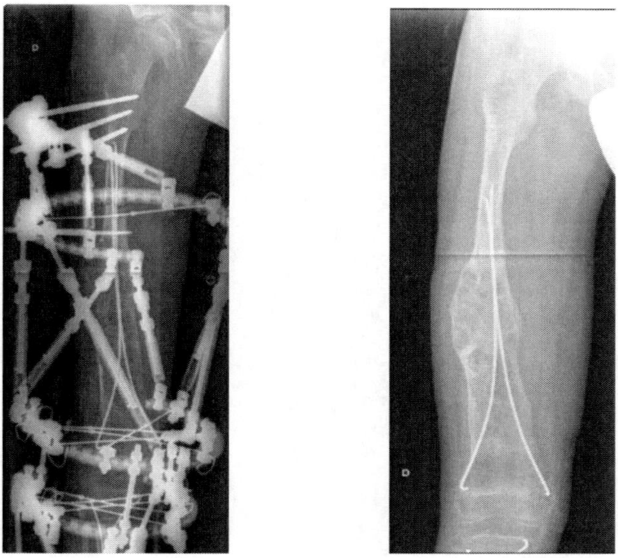

(a) (b)

Figure 18. Use of combined technique of limb lengthening in the patient with fibrous dysplasia: bifocal femoral lengthening and deformity correction by hybrid external fixator (Ilizarov+TSF) associated with FIN (**a**), after frame removal FIN remained in place (**b**).

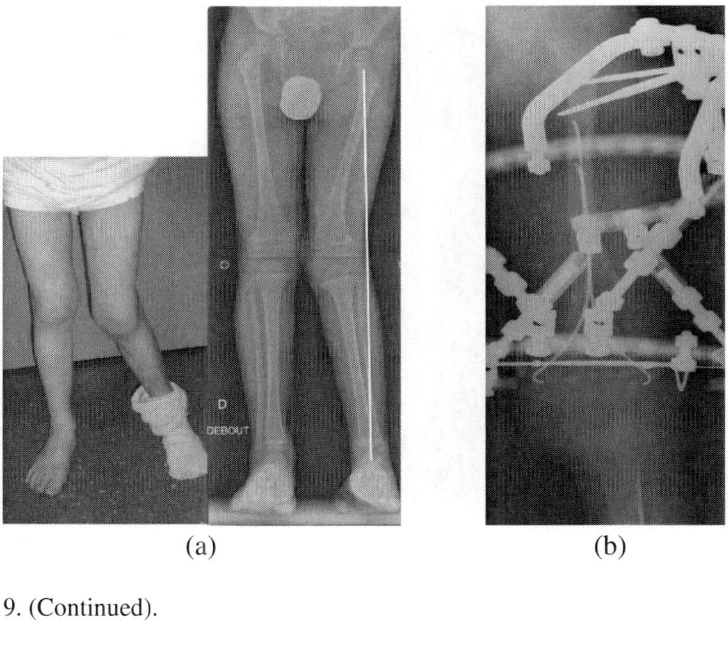

(a) (b)

Figure 19. (Continued).

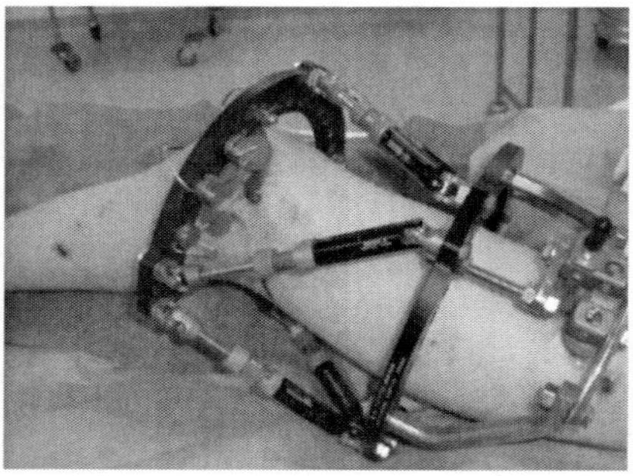

(c)

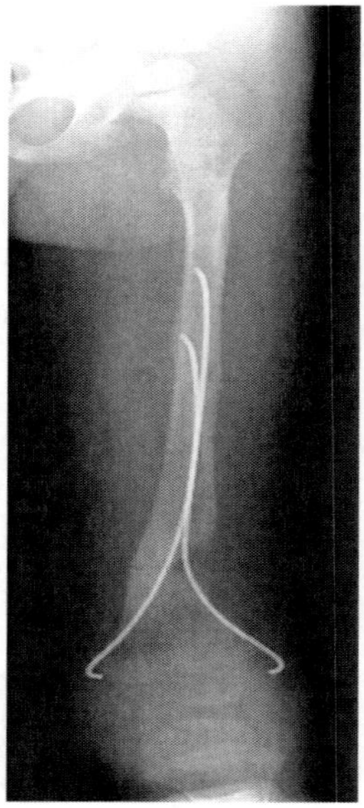

(d)

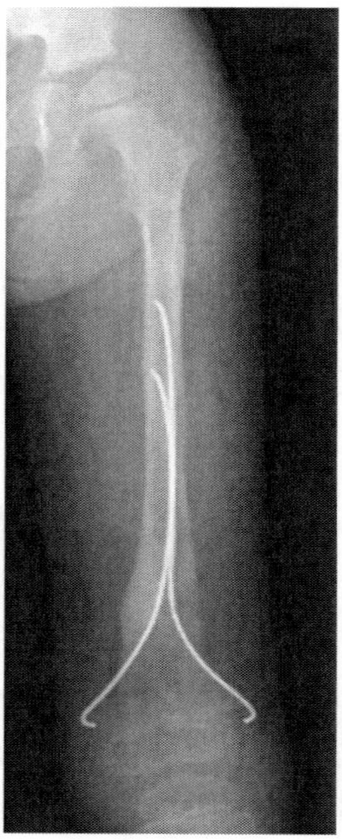

(e)

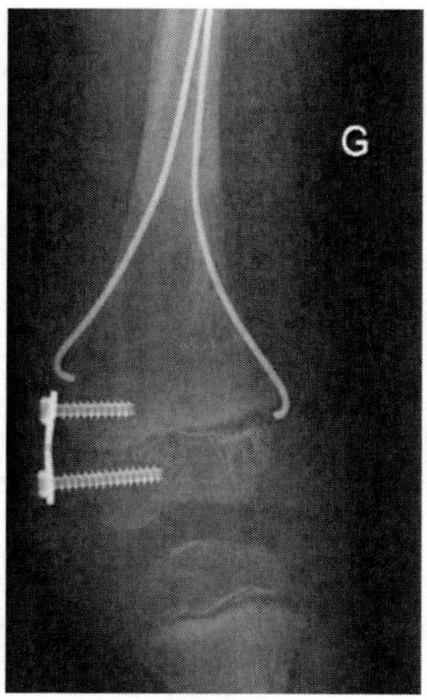

(f)

Figure 19. (Continued).

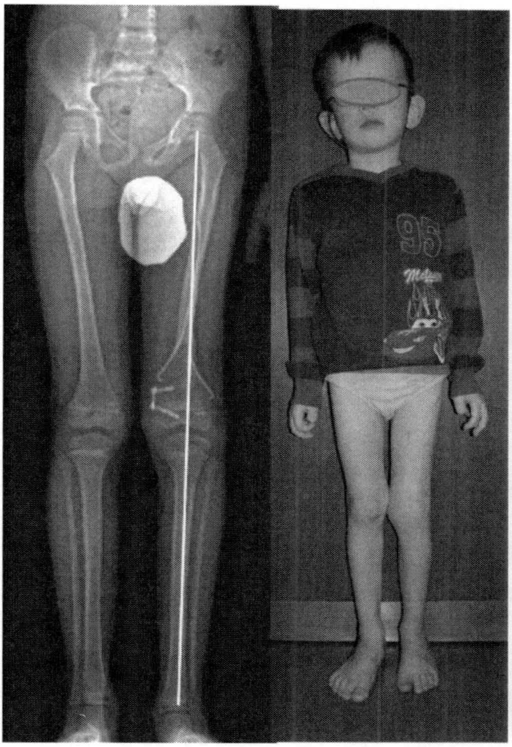

(g)

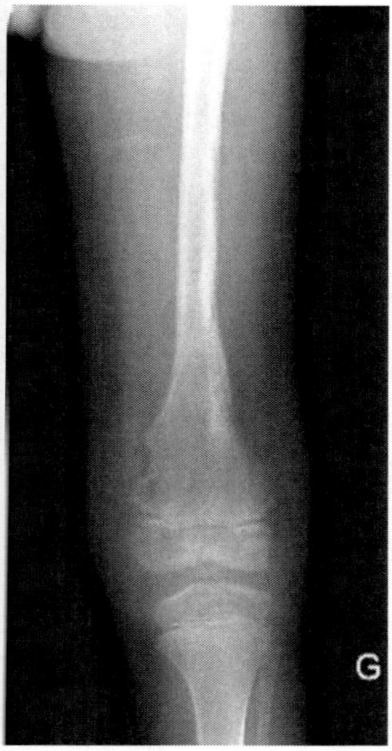

(h)

Figure 19. Patient T., 7 y.o., neurofibromatosis, type I: X-rays of lower limbs and foto of the patient before treatment (**a**), X-rays of the lengthened femur, fixation period (**b**), local infection near two wires in the distal ring caused their removal (**c**), fracture at the level of regenerat in 3 days after frame removal (**d**), bone consolidation obtained with valgus deformity (**e**), internal distal hemiepiphysiodesis by 8-plat (**f**), correction of the valgus deformity achieved in 14 months (**g**), X-rays after plate and FIN removal (**h**).

Discussion

Improvement of bone lengthening procedure by means of external fixation remains topical. The duration of fixator wearing is often long because of the healing index, that makes from 35 days/cm to 65 days/cm according to several publications [7, 16-19]. It may cause multiple complications. Eralp et al. [205] mention the index of 1.65 month/cm in lengthening of the tibia by the Ilizarov fixator, and Sluga et al. [14] in application of the TSF – 48.4 days/cm. The index of consolidation usually obtained by conventional Ilizarov method is 24 to 30 days/cm in femoral or tibial lengthening and 30 to 40 days/cm in the forearm [3].

According to data of Donnan et al. [21] the HI makes 46.4 days/cm in femoral lengthening and 37.3 days/cm in tibial one when applying monolateral fixators of the Orthofix type. After McAndrew et al. [22] – 40.8 days/cm. Besides, the authors mix all the etiologies including achondroplasia, congenital, post-traumatic discrepancy and so on, that we consider unjustified. In some publications analyzing the treatment period one can find the authors' opinion on influence of various factors on the period of consolidation. Thus, Matsubara et al. [5] precise that the HI decreases to 42.5 days/cm in combination of gradual lengthening by the Ilizarov fixator or TSF with the gradual correction of associated deformities in comparison to the acute correction in the beginning of lengthening, when the HI makes 58.6 days/cm. El-Mowafi et al. [23] describe a favourable effect of low-frequency stimulation of bone regeneration with the ultrasound: the HI reduces from 48 to 30 days/cm of lengthening. Finally Kim et al. [4] state that the nailing of a lengthened tibia with a nail of a diameter of 10 mm allowed to decrease the HI to 40.53 days/cm. In simultaneous ipsilateral femoral and tibial lengthening with the Ilizarov method, Curran observed in 4 patients the average femoral healing index of 28 days/cm and the average tibial healing index of 29 days/cm [16].

Besides, some acceleration of treatment can be achieved by different ways [2, 11, 24]. In addition to known methods of lengthening, we propose to unite two methods for the limb lengthening: the gradual distraction with the Ilizarov fixator or TSF and FIN [3, 25]. This combination enables to add certain advantages of the elastic intramedullary nailing to all the improvements of the distraction osteosynthesis.

Our previous comparative studies have shown that the combined technique (circular ExFix+FIN) allows the mean HI reduction of 7 days/cm or to decrease the distraction-consolidation time by 20% in limb lengthening [3, 25].

Other authors also reported this effect of HI reduction using a ring fixator with FIN [7, 8]. Furthermore, accelerated bone consolidation was observed in a short series of femur lengthening, where the monolateral Orthofix fixator was applied with FIN [9].

In contrast to combined methods of distraction osteosynthesis using intramedullary rigid nail [4-6], application of elastic nail reveals an advantage to combine lengthening with progressive deformity (axial and/or rotational) correction. This approach makes additional prealignment procedure unnecessary [3, 25, 26]. The second undisputable advantage of our method is a possibility to perform it in children without any risk to damage the physis. Clearly, an insertion of a rigid nail cannot avoid partial destruction, at least, of one growth zone.

Besides, the benefit of a reduced HI is a low rate of complications. We observed a significant decrease, even absence of those complications which are caused by long distraction-consolidation delay: pin/wire site infection, joint stiffness, hemorrhagic complications at pin site, as well as complications caused by low rate of bone regeneration: delayed consolidation (HI superior to 45 days/cm), deformity or fracture after frame removal [17, 27-29]. FIN left in situ allowed to minimize and even eradicate such specific problems as pathologic fractures at the level of fibrous or cartilaginous zone in our series of patients presenting diseases associated with bony fragility (fibrous dysplasia, Ollier disease) [30, 31].

So, the demonstrated and prooved advantages of the combined method for limb lengthening (ExFix+FIN) are reduction of HI, low rate of septic, articular and bony complications, prevention of pathologic fractures. Finally, we observed the good and excellent results in 93.5% of cases in this series.

The results are scored as good or excellent only if the planned length gain was achieved, planned duration of treatment was respected, there was no any complication impairing functional outcome, e.g. without sequelae.

It is worth of mentioning that only perfect performing of FIN associated with the Ilizarov fixator allows to respect all the obligatory conditions of the distraction osteosynthesis (Ilizarov method), namely, preservation of the bone surrounding, periosteum and especially intramedullary vascularization, respecting of biological rates of lengthening, preservation of the function by an early articular mobilization and weight bearing, respecting certain biomechanical rules. So, all the conditions are united in a way that enables association of indisputable advantages of FIN with the Ilizarov method of lengthening by means of the Ilizarov frame itself or TSF. Nevertheless, the result depends first of all on the personal experience of the surgeon in both the limb lengthening technique and the flexible intramedullary nailing [3, 25].

CONCLUSION

The flexible intramedullary nailing, a low invasive and elegant method, allows to add multiple advantages to the method of limb lengthening with the external fixator. This combination seems to us well proved and logic. FIN, when correctly applied, respects the bone biological features which are essential for successful limb lengthening. The major effect of application of the combination of external circular fixation with FIN is a significant decrease of duration of the external osteosynthesis.

REFERENCES

[1] Gubin AV, Borzunov DY, Malkova TA (2013) The Ilizarov paradigm: thirty years with the Ilizarov method, current concerns and future research. *Int Orthop.* 37(8):1533-1539.

[2] Shevtsov VI, Popkov AV, Popkov DA, Prevot J (2001) Réduction de la durée du traitement dans les allongements osseux progressifs. *Rev Chir Orthop.* 87:248-256.

[3] Popkov D, Popkov A, Haumont Th, Journeau P, Lascombes P (2010) Flexible intramedullary nail use in limb lengthening. *J Pediatr Orthop.* 30:910-918.

[4] Kim H, Lee SK, Kim KJ, et al. (2009) Tibial lengthening using a reamed type intramedullary nail and an Ilizarov external fixator. *Int Orthop.* 33:835–841.

[5] Matsubara H, Tsuchiya H, Sakurakichi K, Watanabe K, Tomita K (2006) Deformity correction and lengthening of lower legs with an external fixator. *International orthopaedics.* 30 (6): 550-554.

[6] Paley D, Herzenberg JE, Paremain G, et al. (1997) Femoral lengthening over an intramedullary nail. A matched-case comparison with Ilizarov femoral lengthening. *J Bone Joint Surg Am.* 79:1464–1480.

[7] Launay F, Jouve JL, Guillaume E, Viehweger, Jacquemier M, Bollini G (2001) Les allongements progressifs de l'avant-bras chez l'enfant. A propos d'une série de 14 cas. *Rev Chir Orthop.*87:786-795.

[8] Bukva B, Brdar R, Nikolic D, Petronic I, Ducic S, Abramovic D (2013) Combined external fixation and intramedullary alignment in correction of limb length discrepancies. *Acta Orthop Belg.* 79(4):411-416.

[9] Lampasi M, Launay F, Jouve JL, Bollini G (2009) Femoral lengthening over elastic stable intramedullary nailing in children using the monolateral external fixator. *Chir Organi Mov.* 93(2): 57-64.

[10] Ilizarov GA (1990) Clinical application of the tension-stress effect for limb lengthening. *Clin. Orthop.* 250:8-26.

[11] Ilizarov GA (1992) *Transosseous ostheosynthesis*, Berlin: Springer-Verlag.

[12] Paley D, Herzenberg JE, Tetsworth K, McKie J, Bhave A (1994) Deformity planning for frontal and sagittal plane corrective osteotomies. *Orthop Clin North Am.*3:425-465.

[13] Paley D. Correction of limb deformities in the 21st century (2000) *J Pediatr Orthop.* 20:279-281.

[14] Sluga M, Pfeiffer M, Kotz R, Nehrer S (2003) Lower limb deformities in children: two-stage correction using Taylor spatial frame. *J Pediatr Orthop* B. 12:123-128.

[15] Lascombes P, Popkov D, Huber H, Haumont T, Journeau P (2012) Classification of complications after progressive long bone lengthening: proposal for a new classification. *Orthop Traumatol Surg Res.* 98(6):629-637.

[16] Curran AR, Kuo KN, Lubicky JP (1999) Silmultaneous ipsilateral femoral and tibial lengthening with the Ilizarov method. *J Pediatr Orthop.* 19:386-390.

[17] Glorion C, Pouliquen JC, Langlais J, Ceolin JL, Kassis B (1995) Allongement de fémur par callotasis. Etude d'une série de 79 cas chez l'enfant et l'adolescent. *Rev Chir Orthop.* 81:147-156.

[18] Song HR, Myrboh V, Oh CW, Lee ST, Lee SH (2005) Tibial lengthening and concomitant foot deformity correction in 14 patients with permanent deformity after poliomyelitis. *Acta Orthop.* 76 (2):261-269.

[19] Stanitski DF, Shahcheraghi H, Nicker DA, Armstrong PF (1996) Results of tibial lengthening with the Ilizarov technique. *J Pediatr Orthop.* 16:168-172.

[20] Eralp L, Kocaoğlu M, Ozkan K, Türker M (2004) A comparison of two osteotomy techniques for tibial lengthening. *Archives of orthopaedic and trauma surgery.* 124 (5): 298-300.

[21] Donnan LT, Saleh M, Rigby AS (2003) Acute correction of lower limb deformity and simultaneous lengthening with a monolateral fixator *JBJS* (B). 85:254-260.

[22] McAndrew AR, Saleh M (2007) Limb lengthening by Villarubias method: the Sheffield Children's Hospital experience. *J Pediatr Orthop* B. 16:233-235.

[23] El-Mowafi H, Mohsen M (2005) The effect of low-intensity pulsed ultrasound on callus maturation in tibial distraction osteogenesis. *Int Orthop.* 29(2):121-124.

[24] Shevtsov VI, Popkov AV (1995) Automatic distractional osteosynthesis. *Hospital Management International.* 265-269.

[25] Lascombes P (2010) *Flexible intramedullary nailing in children.* Berlin Heidelberg: Springer-Verlag.

[26] Popkov D, Lascombes P, Popkov A, Journeau P, Haumont T (2012) Role of the flexible intramedullary nailing in limb lengthening in children: comparative study based on the series of 295 lengthenins. *Europ Orthop Traum.* 3:17-24.

[27] Popkov AV (1991) Errors and complications of operative lengthening of the lower extremities in adults by the Ilizarov method. *Vestn Khir I I Grek.* 1:113-116.

[28] Rybka V, Richtr M (1989) The index of relative prolongation in leg lengthening. *Min Orthop Traumatol.* 40:443-444.

[29] Launay F, Younsi R, Pithioux M, Chabrand P, Bollini G, Jouve JL (2013) Fracture following lower limb lengthening in children: a series of 58 patients. *Orthop Traumatol Surg Res.*99(1):72-79.

[30] Jesus-Garcia R, Bongiovanni JC, Korukian M, Boatto H, Seixas MT, Laredo J (2001). Use of the Ilizarov external fixator in the treatment of patients with Ollier's disease. *Clin Orthop Relat Res.* 382:82-86.

[31] Popkov D, Journeau P, Popkov A, Haumont T, Lascombes P (2010) Ollier's disease limb lenghtening: Should intramedullary nailing be combined with circular external fixation? *Orthop Traumatol Surg Res.* 96:348-353.

In: Combined Stimulating Methods …
Editor: Dmitry Popkov
ISBN: 978-1-63483-028-7

Chapter IV

Influence of Lengthening on the Residual Limb Growth

***Pierre Journeau*[1], *Dmitry Popkov*[2*] and *Pierre Lascombes*[3]**

[1]Pediatric Orthopedic Surgery Dept, Nancy University Hospital Center, Children's Hospital, Vandoeuvre, France
[2]Scientific and Clinical Laboratory for Deformity Correction and Limb Lengthening, Federal Russian State-Financed Ilizarov Scientific Center for Restorative Traumatology and Orthopaedics, Kurgan, Russia
[3]Pediatric Orthopedic Surgery Dept, Geneva University Hospitals, Children's Hospital, Geneva, Switzerland

Abstract

Introduction. Prognosis of limb length discrepancy in children affected by congenital abnormality remains a subject of concern. Therapeutic strategy must take length prediction into account in order to adapt equalization techniques and the timing of treatment. Initial prognosis, however, may need revising after completion of one or several surgical interventions on the pathologic limb.

* Corresponding author: Ilizarov Scientific Center for Restorative Traumatology and Orthopaedics, 6, M.-Ulyanova Street, 640014 Kurgan, Russia; dpopkov@mail.ru.

The aim of this study was to determine different types of growth response that a bone segment can present after progressive lengthening in case of congenital limb length discrepancy.

Materials and methods. Treatment results were analyzed in 150 patients with congenital lower limb length discrepancy, who underwent surgery at age from 2 to 15 years old. Bone segment growth rates were measured before lengthening, during the first year after frame removal and, finally, over long-term follow-up, calculating the ratios of radiological bone length to the number of months between two measurements. Mean follow-up was 5.1±1.3 years.

Results. Changes in short- and long-term growth rate distinguished five patterns of bone behavior after lengthening, ranging from growth acceleration to total inhibition.

Discussion and Conclusion. These five residual growth patterns depended on certain factors causing acceleration or, on the contrary, slowing down of growth: age at the lengthening surgery, percentage of lengthening and minimal period between two lengthenings. These criteria help to optimize conditions for resumed growth after progressive segmental lengthening, avoiding conditions liable to induce slowing down or inhibition, and providing a planning aid in multi-step lengthening programs.

Keywords: Congenital lower limb length discrepancy, bone lengthening, residual growth

INTRODUCTION

One of the major issues of the long-term follow up after limb lengthening remains the change of longitudinal growth function of the operated segment.

Residual growth after progressive lengthening has been the focus of several studies [1-9], but the evolution of congenital lower-limb length discrepancy in children undergoing progressive lengthening remains unforeseeable and the factors relevant to bone segment activity in these cases remain undetermined. Both slowing and boosted growth patterns have been reported, independently of the lengthening technique employed (Judet, Wagner, Callotasis or Cauchoix) [2-6], other authors finding no change in growth rates [7-9].

The present retrospective study sought to identify factors affecting residual growth after progressive lengthening: age at lengthening, percentage of lengthening, and single- or multistep strategy.

MATERIAL AND METHODS

We studied outcomes in 150 patients with congenital unilateral limb length discrepancy (girls/boys=79/71), to whom Ilizarov lower limb lengthening was performed at age from 2 to 15 years old (the average 8.3±2.9 years old). The series was homogeneous for etiology and surgical procedure. In total the patients underwent 207 stages of surgical segment lengthening. In 42 cases the segment was lengthened twice and in 15 – thrice.

Femoral lengthening gain ranged from 1.5 to 7 cm reaching the average of 4.2±1.43 cm or 17.3%±12.18% of the initial segment length. The index of fixation ranged from 2 to 47.3 days/cm (the mean 15.2±12.03 days/cm), the healing index – from 11.8 d/cm to 66 d/cm (the average 29.9±17.56 d/cm)

Tibial lengthening gain ranged from 2 to 7 cm reaching the average of 4.8±2.38 cm or 19.3%±11.04% of the initial segment length. The index of fixation ranged from 3.3 to 44.3 d/cm (the mean 15.7±10.41 d/cm), the healing index – from 10 to 73.3 d/cm (the average 28.6±13.0 d/cm).

In this series of patients the natural growth of a shortened limb was assessed before surgical treatment, in 1-3, 6-8, 9-12 months after the treatment and during 3-7 years of the long-term follow up.

Hechard-Carlioz charts [10] were used for monitoring femoral and tibial longitudinal growth. Preoperatively, predicted limb-length discrepancy and final segment length were assessed with multiplier method [11] taking into account that, without treatment, the natural growth of a malformed segment is linear, with a constant rate, so that change in percentage discrepancy will likewise be linear [12].

To investigate possible growth-rate change after lengthening, whether stimulation, transitory slowing of growth during the first year or definitive cessation of growth, the following index was calculated at end of growth phase:

$$RGG\ (\%) = (PFSSD - (LG \pm FRSD)) \times 100\% \ / \ FLSL$$

where: RGG = residual growth gain; PFSSD = predicted final spontaneous segmental discrepancy (mm); LG = length gain achieved by external fixation (mm); FRSD = final residual segmental discrepancy (mm: healthy segment length minus lengthened segment length); and FLSL = final lengthened segment length (mm).

This index represents the change in spontaneous growth after progressive lengthening with respect to the final length of the lengthened segment; it may be positive (growth stimulation), neutral (no change) or negative (slowing of spontaneous growth).

Results

Observing the longitudinal growth we distinguished the following types of change of the growth rate of the operated segment in short and long-term follow up.

Type I – increased growth rate by the end of lengthening progressively decreasing by the 9-12th month after the end of treatment, but the growth rate remains higher than initial during the long-term follow up (Figures 20, 24 and 25).

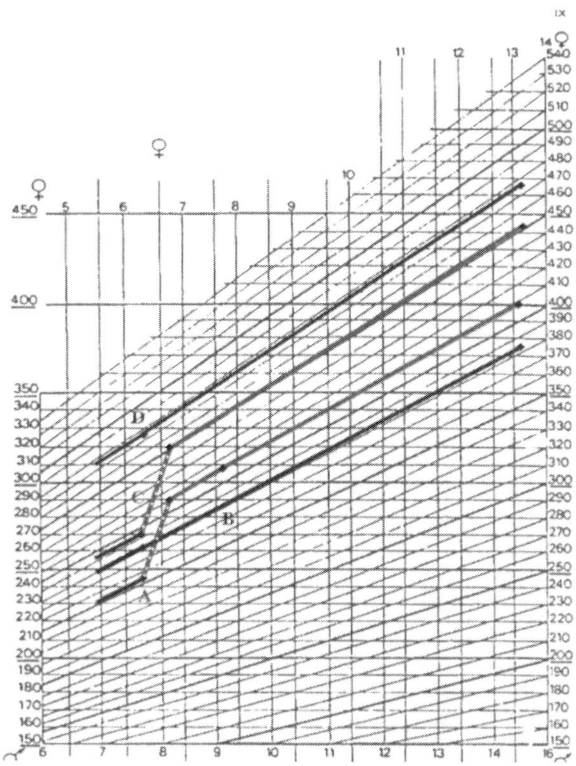

Figure 20. Diagram of segment growth (dotted line corresponds to bone lengthening, A – growth of short tibia, B – growth of normal tibia, C – growth of short femur, D – growth of normal femur): type I of residual growth of lengthened segments.

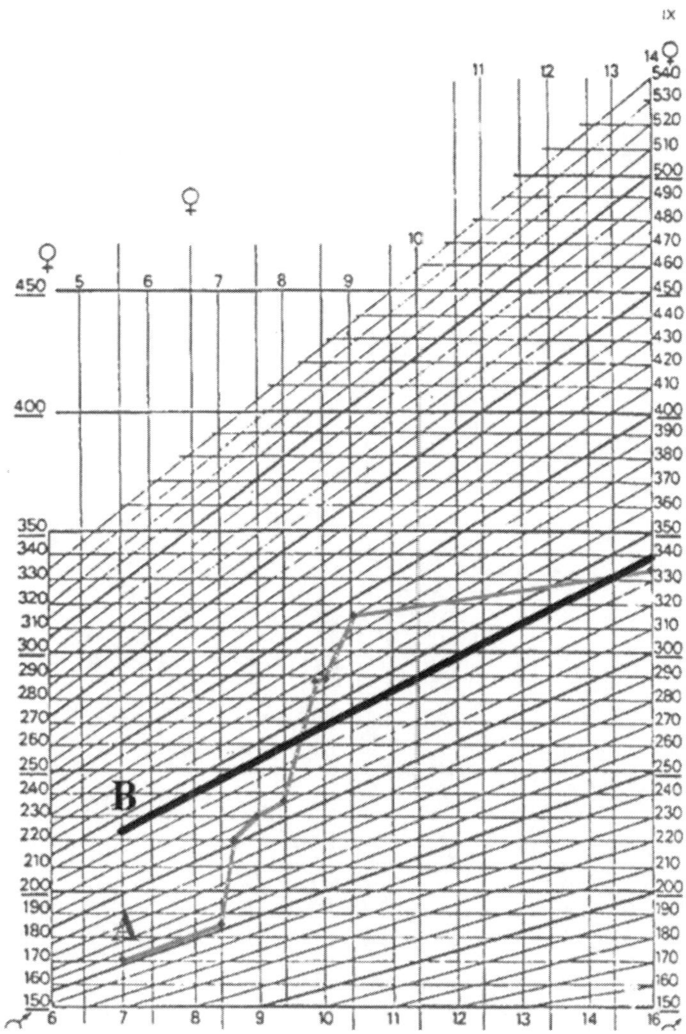

Figure 21. Diagram of segment growth (dotted line corresponds to bone lengthening, A – growth of short tibia, B – growth of normal tibia, C – growth of short femur, D – growth of normal femur): type II of residual growth after the first lengthening, type V after iterative lengthening.

Type II - increased growth rate returning to the initial one by the 9-12th month after frame removal. In the long-term follow up the growth rate is close to preoperative (Figure 21).

Type III – growth rate increase is observed during the first postoperative year but in the long-term follow up the growth rate is slower than initial (Figure 22).

Type IV – immediate inhibition or absence of longitudinal growth of the segment is observed till the 6-8th month after the end of surgical lengthening followed by returning to the initial growth rate (Figure 23).

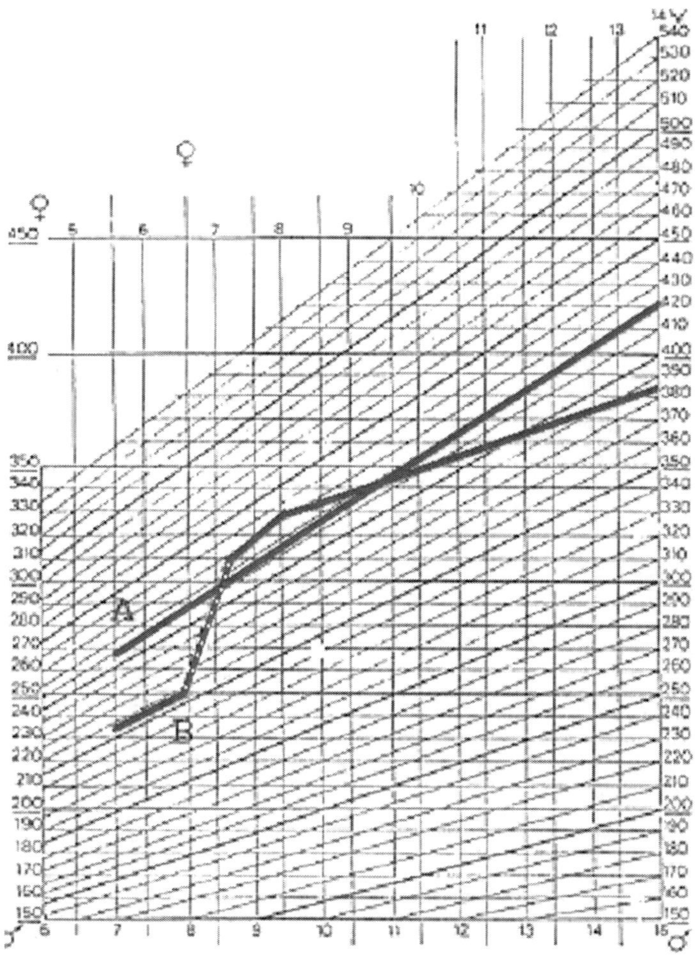

Figure 22. Diagram of segment growth (dotted line corresponds to bone lengthening, A – growth of normal tibia, B – growth of short tibia): type III of the residual growth.

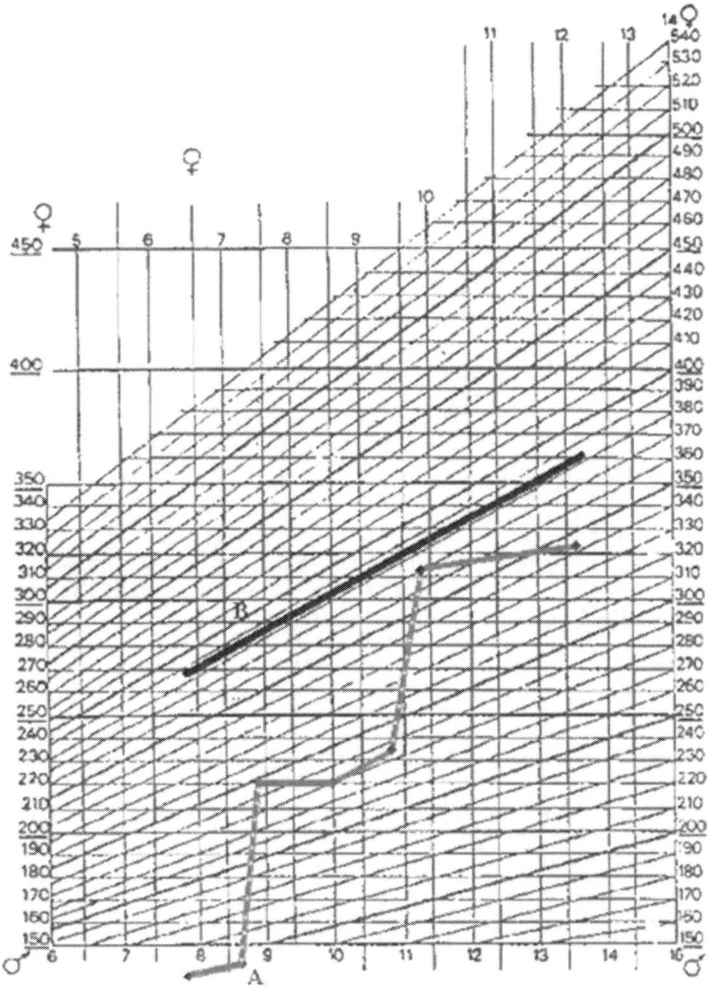

Figure 23. Diagram of segment growth (dotted line corresponds to bone lengthening, A – growth of short tibia, B - growth of normal tibia): type IV of the residual growth after the first lengthening, Type V – after iterative lengthening.

Type V – progressive decrease of the growth rate after the treatment down to full stop for several months followed by stabilization of the growth rate at values inferior to initial (Figure 23).

Tables IV.1 and IV.2 demonstrate change of the mean growth rate of lengthened femur and tibia in various groups of patients.

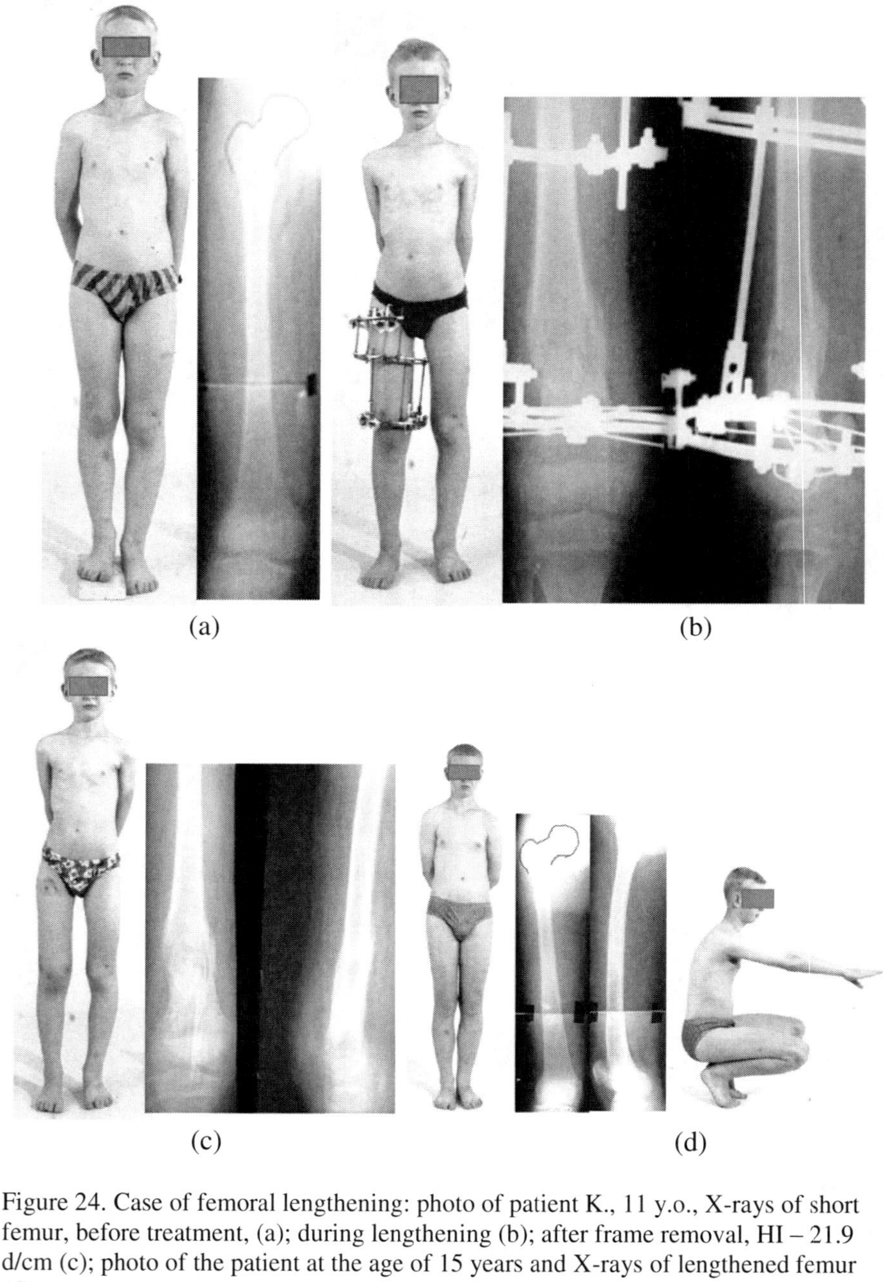

Figure 24. Case of femoral lengthening: photo of patient K., 11 y.o., X-rays of short femur, before treatment, (a); during lengthening (b); after frame removal, HI – 21.9 d/cm (c); photo of the patient at the age of 15 years and X-rays of lengthened femur (d).

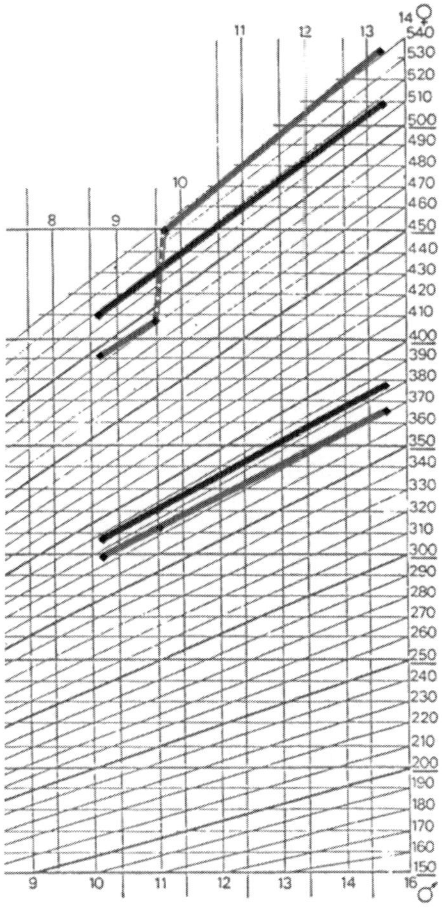

Figure 25. Diagram of the segment growth of the patient K (from Figure 24).

Table IV.1. The mean values of growth rate in lengthened femur at different periods of observation

Groups of patients according to the growth type	Femoral growth rate at different periods of observation; mm/month				
	Before surgery	2-3 months	6-8 months	9-12 months	Long-term follow up
I	1.38±0.47	3.05±1.84	2.8±0.86	2.3±0.94	1.6±0.60
II	1.35±0.20	1.53±0.41	1.36±1.19	1.3±0.21	1.37±0.10
III	1.4±0.33	1.59±0.29	1.3±0.37	1.15±0.62	0.9±0.20
IV	1.26±0.30	0.22±0.37	0.55±0.48	2.03±1.02	1.8±0.64
V	1.27±0.74	0.43±0.62	0.33±0.58	0.42±0.40	0.24±0.65

Table IV.2. The mean values of growth rate in lengthened tibia at different periods of observation

Groups of patients according to the growth type	Tibial growth rate at different periods of observation; mm/month				
	Before surgery	2-3 months	6-8 months	9-12 months	Long-term follow up
I	1.13±0.29	2.6±0.96	1.51±0.68	1.8±0.53	1.48±0.27
II	1.24±0.31	2.7±2.03	-	1.25±0.25	1.25±0.35
III	1.1±0.46	3.7±2.43	2.1±0.56	0.76±0.37	0.73±0.28
IV	1.16±0.30	0.21±0.32	1.20±1.56	1.3±1.29	1.7±0.48
V	1.18±0.50	0.34±0.49	0.4±0.42	0.43±0.43	0.6±0.40

Comparing various groups to each other according to the relative amount of lengthening and healing index, no statistically significant difference was found. Choice of a method for femoral or tibial lengthening also had no significant influence on change of the following growth type. Distribution of cases between the groups of patients is of a proportional character. Reconstructive surgery on foot bones is of a great importance whether performed simultaneously with tibial lengthening or during the long-term follow up. In such cases the tibial growth rate is slower than initial. This correlation was noticed even in the primary lengthening: two patients with growth rate of type II and III and four patients with type V.

Comparison of group I and group V according to the data presented in table IV.3 allows the statement that second and third stage of femoral lengthening necessitates inhibition of a natural segment growth. On the other hand, it is the primary surgical lengthening of the segment that stimulates the following growth.

Table IV.3. Distribution of femoral growth types according to the stage of lengthening; number of observations

Growth type	Primary lengthening	Second lengthening	Third lengthening
I	49	1	0
II	18	0	0
III	12	3	0
IV	5	0	0
V	6	20	7

Table IV.4. Distribution of tibial growth types according to the stage of lengthening; number of observations

Growth type	Primary lengthening	Second lengthening	Third lengthening
I	59	0	0
II	21	2	2
III	5	0	0
IV	11	4	0
V	8	24	11

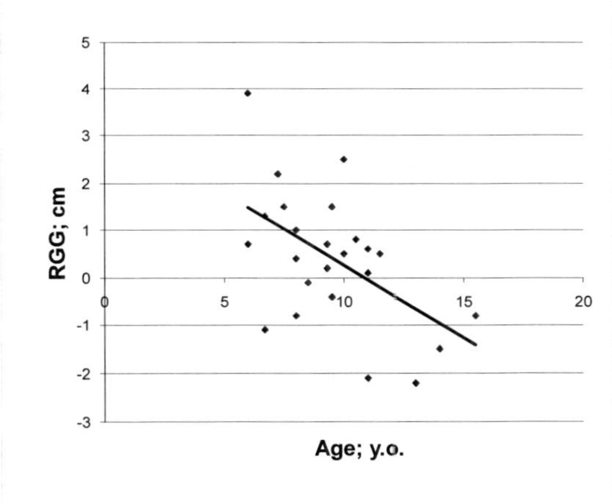

(a)

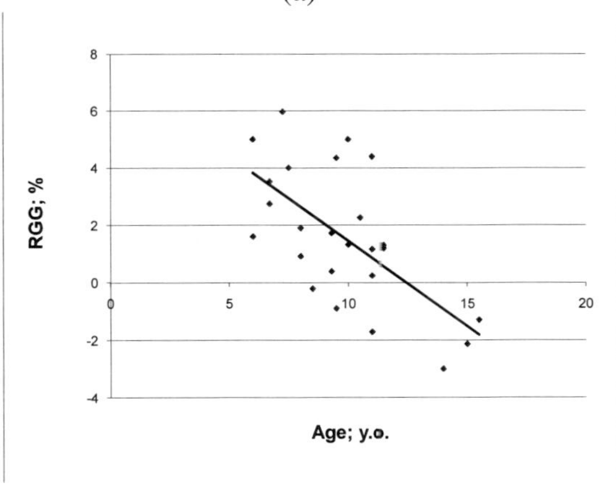

(b)

Figure 26. Relations between RGG (in boys) and age of lengthening, in cm (a) and % (b).

In tibial lengthening we also observed inhibition of natural growth after consecutive lengthening (Table IV.4). After primary lengthening the decrease of longitudinal growth rate was noticed in presence of severe malformation of a proximal femur or if the lengthening was performed at age of 13-15 years old, i.e. prior to the end of natural growth. Reconstructive osteotomies on foot bones in 4 cases were associated with inhibition of longitudinal tibial growth in the long-term follow up even after the first lengthening.

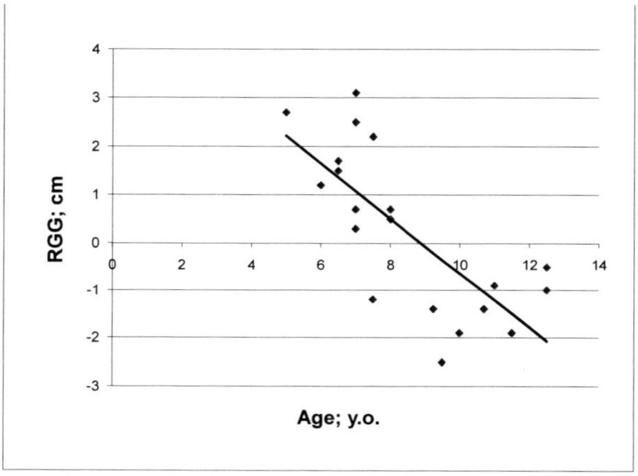

(a)

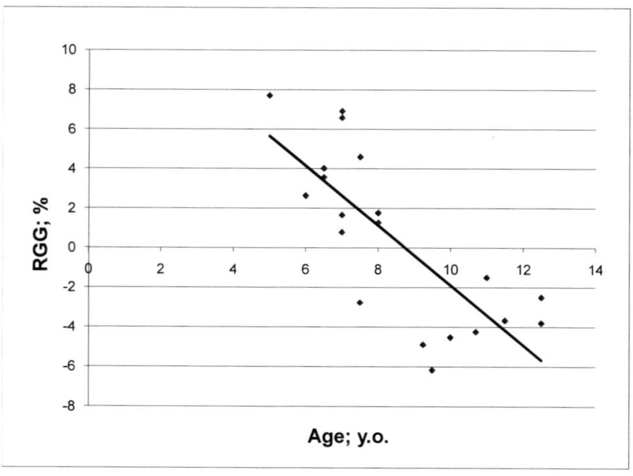

(b)

Figure 27. Relations between RGG (in girls) and age of lengthening, in cm (a) and % (b).

Figures 26 and 27 shows correlation between the age at the beginning of treatment and residual growth gain in the first stage of lower limb lengthening. Since the bone age of 8.5-9 years in girls and 12 years in boys the stimulation of longitudinal growth of the lengthened segment is not observed.

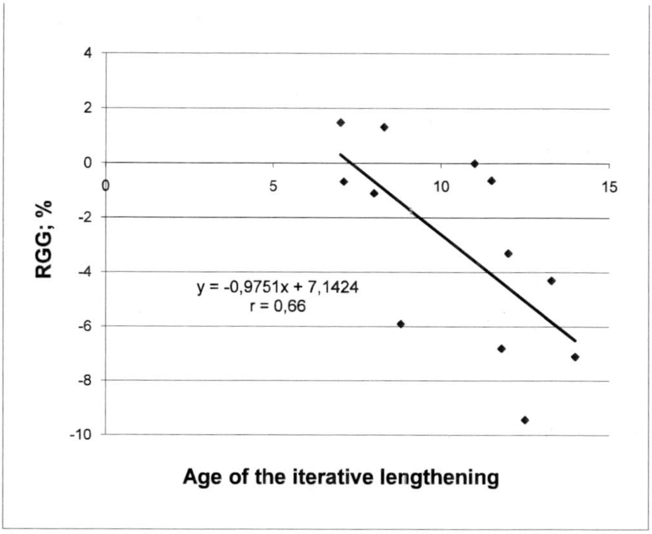

(a)

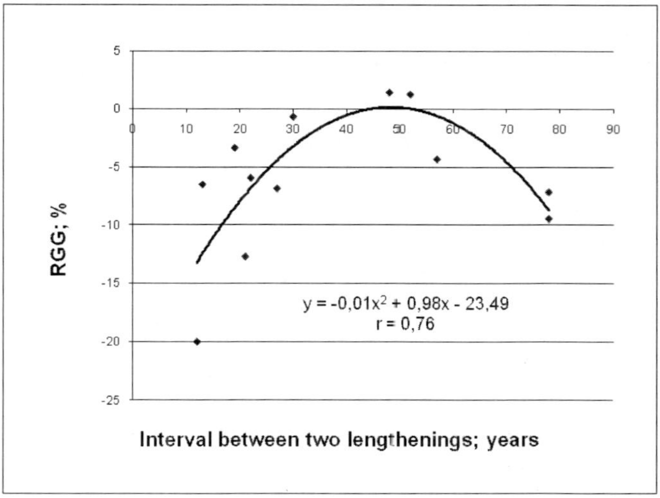

(b)

Figure 28. Relations between RGG and age of iterative lengthening (a) or RGG and delay between two lengthenings of the same segment (b).

Besides, the age at the beginning of the second stage of lengthening and delay between stages are important for the following growth of segment. Figure 28 demonstrates influence of the age at the beginning of the second stage of lengthening and the time period between the stages on the following longitudinal growth of segment.

According to the above mentioned data it is obvious that in order to prevent the inhibition of the following growth, the second stage of lengthening should be performed before prepubertal growth acceleration and the most favorable delay between the lengthening stages of the same segment is about four years.

If the same segment was lengthened trice, all patients manifested inhibition of longitudinal growth with negative value of residual growth gain. Absolute length loss was 5.0±1.27 cm, relative – 11.9±2.84%. Thereat, total amount of lengthening in femur was 15±2.25cm and in tibia – 13.8±1.92 cm. Thus, triple lengthening of a segment during the period of natural growth is considered inexpedient.

DISCUSSION

In congenital lower-limb length discrepancy, lengthening procedures often need to be performed before the end of spontaneous growth, due to the functional and psychological impact of the discrepancy on child and family. Prognosis of the growth of an operated limb is an important component of lengthening strategy.

The present series exclusively included congenital pathology, making it homogeneous. As congenital discrepancies show a percentage length difference that remains stable over growth in absence of treatment, we accepted the hypothesis that any observed change in growth pattern would be identical across all congenital etiologies, independently of segment location.

Growth stimulation following a first Ilizarov lengthening procedure was systematic when bone age was less than 12 years in boys or 9 years in girls.

This mechanism may be explained by stimulation due to increased vascularization during lengthening, or by a mechanical cause [5]. Some reports stressed the importance of having a correct biomechanical axis and of functional loading to minimize disturbance of conjunctive cartilage growth over periods exceeding 2 years [13,14]. Experimental studies showed that cell number per column in the growth area depends on the forces acting on the cartilage, increasing with increased loading. The greater the number of cells, the more active the cartilage [15]. Antonov demonstrated the growth-stimulating effect of functional forces under dynamic loading [13]. Absence of functional weight-bearing can slow down the longitudinal growth. It explains inhibition of tibial growth while reconstructive surgeries on foot simultaneously with tibial lengthening. External fixation allows all deformities to be progressively corrected, avoiding impairment of joint range of motion during lengthening and ensuring a perfect biomechanical axis in three dimensions [16-18].

Penneçot et al. [2] reported a significant impact on the growth plate after progressive bone lengthening by Judet distractor. The harmful effects of hyperpressure on the conjunctive cartilage, impaired vascularization and the resultant shaft ischemia may account for subsequent slowing of growth. However, the 1-2 mm initial joint-line distraction reported by Oostenbroek et al. was probably insufficient to prevent contact between the joint surfaces and avoid shaft compression [19]. Joint bridging avoids inducing subluxation and hyperpressure threatening the conjunctive cartilage. In the present series, there was no significant difference in residual growth rate associated with bridging of the knee, and no conclusion can thus be drawn as to whether bridging, performed basically to avoid joint impairment, also protects the tibial shaft.

The reduction in growth observed, however, was not necessarily related to the hyperpressure effects described by the above authors. Obtaining and maintaining a normal axis during the lengthening procedure seems to us to be a necessary but not sufficient condition for growth to be conserved.

Percentage lengthenings emerged as one of the main factors impacting residual growth. An experimental study, however, reported that a lengthening of 30% did not affect longitudinal tibial growth [20]; these conclusions were drawn from morphological results at only 5 weeks' follow up. Clinical data, in contrast, demonstrate the negative impact of such a length gain. Viehweger et al. [6], in series of 34 children, reported a clear impact on residual growth following lengthening exceeding 30% using a unilateral external fixator. One of our studies [21] demonstrates that single-step lengthening of more than 30% of initial segment length is to be avoided in congenital lower-limb length discrepancy, as it may impair resumption of growth.

Osseous age at time of lengthening is a factor to be taken into account in treatment planning in congenital lower-limb abnormality. Pouliquen et al. [3] reported that lengthening performed before the age of 11 years induced growth disorder; this series, however, included only six children with congenital discrepancy. The present results, on the contrary, showed greater growth stimulation gain in children aged less than 8 years at time of procedure. These findings are in agreement with those of Suva et al. [5], who reported accelerated growth of a mean 2.5% in all children treated at less than 6 years of age.

In our study has shown that lengthening performed after the start of the pubertal growth boost (here taken as after 12 years' bone age in boys and 10 in girls, due to the impossibility of having a reliable physiological estimate of pubertal maturity) led to a negative RGG and all the more so in the early phases of puberty.

The exact mechanism of slowed growth can only be guessed at. During the intense pubertal spontaneous growth phase, the soft tissue of the lengthened segment cannot adapt to the change in length, which may result in hyper pressure on the growth plate. Suva et al. [5] suggest a phenomenon of growth capital exhaustion to account for slowing.

It also emerged that iterative lengthening of the affected segment induced negative RGG when conducted at close intervals (of less than 3 years). These findings may guide planning length equalization when the discrepancy prognosis requires iterative lengthening: iterative lengthening of a segment should be undertaken before the beginning of the pubertal growth boost but more than 3 years after the first procedure. The alternative is to perform the second lengthening around the end of spontaneous growth. This program can thus be applied to manage severe femoral or tibial hypoplasia.

CONCLUSION

Our results prove that the primary lengthening of lower limb segments in congenital length discrepancy, which is performed before the prepubertal growth acceleration, can be a factor stimulating the following natural growth.

The second stage of lengthening of the segment leads to inhibition of growth of the operated segment. The least inhibition is noted when the delay between two stages of lengthening of the same segment is about 4 years. Another unfavorable factor is performance of reconstructive surgeries on foot both simultaneously with tibial lengthening and during the long-term follow up.

Triple lengthening of the segment during the natural growth should not be performed at all.

All these data should be considered while planning the strategy of surgical treatment of children with congenital lower limb length discrepancy.

References

[1] Dutoit M, Rigault P, Padovani JP, Finidori J, Touzet P, Durand Y (1990) The fate of children undergoing bone lengthening in congenital hypoplasia of the legs. *Rev Chir Orthop.* 76:1-7.

[2] Penneçot GF, Herman S, Pouliquen JC (1983). Effects of progressive lengthening on the growth cartilage. Value of measurement of the torque. *Rev Chir Orthop.* 69:623-627.

[3] 3 Pouliquen JC, Beneux J, Mener G, Penneçot GF (1979) Etude de la croissance du membre inférieur après allongement segmentaire chez l'enfant. *Ann Orthop Ouest.* 11:95-98.

[4] Sharma M, MacKenzie WG, Bowen JR (1996) Severe tibial growth retardation in total fibular hemimelia after limb lengthening. *J Pediatr Orthop.* 16:438-444.

[5] Suva D, Naccarato LH, Heripret G, Cauchoix J, Morel G (1984) An unknown after surgical lengthening of the femur in children: spontaneous postoperative parasitic lengthening. *Rev Chir Orthop.* 70:631-636.

[6] Viehweger E, Pouliquen JC, Kassis B (1998) Bone growth after lengthening of the lower limb in children. *J Pediatr Orthop B.* 7:154-157.

[7] Hope PG, Crawfurd EJ, Catterall A (1994) Bone growth following lengthening for congenital shortening of the lower limb. *J Pediatr Orthop.* 14:339-342.

[8] Sabharwal S, Paley D, Bhave A, Herzenberg JE (2000) Growth patterns after lengthening of congenitally short lower limbs in young children. *J Pediatr Orthop.* 20:137-145.

[9] McCarthy JJ, Kim H, Saluan P, Karsky D, Davidson RS (2003) The effects of limb lengthening on growth. *J Pediatr Orthop B.*12:328-331.

[10] Hechard P, Carlioz H (1978) Practical method of prediction of leg length inequality. *Rev Chir Orthop.* 64:81-87.

[11] Paley D, Bhave A, Herzenberg JE, Bowen JR (2000) Multiplier method for predicting limb-length discrepancy. *J Bone Joint Surg.* 82-A:1432-1446.

[12] Shapiro F (1982) Developmental patterns in lower-extremity length discrepancies. *J Bone Joint Surg.* 64-Am:639-651.

[13] Antonov SG (1979) Effect of physical loading on the state of the metaepiphyseal cartilage of the femoral bones and on the growth of these bones in length. *Arkh Anat Histol Embriol.* 76:75-81.

[14] Chargorodsky VS, Iljin LA (1972) Distribution of tension at the level of distal femoral physics. *Orthop Traum Protez.*1:33-38.

[15] Damsin JP, Djenadi K, Josset P, Wioland M (1996) Cartilage de croissance et croissance en orthopédie. *EMC Appareil locomoteur.* 14-009-A-10:13.

[16] Popkov D, Popkov A, Haumont Th, Journeau P, Lascombes P (2010) Flexible intramedullary nail use in limb lengthening. *J Pediatr Orthop.* 30:910-918.

[17] Catagni MA, Radwan M, Lovisetti L, Guerreschi F, Elmoghazy NA (2011) Limb lengthening and deformity correction by the Ilizarov technique in type III fibular hemimelia: an alternative to amputation. *Clin Orthop Relat Res.* 469(4):1175-1180.

[18] Hamdy RC, Makhdom AM, Saran N, Birch J (2014) Congenital fibular deficiency. *J Am Acad Orthop Surg.* 22(4):246-55.

[19] Oostenbroek HJ, Brand R, Van Roermund PM (2009) Growth rate after limb deformity correction by the Ilizarov method with or without knee joint distraction. Lengthening in 30 children followed for at least 2 years. *Acta Orthop.* 80:338-343.

[20] Gang C, Coulton L, Lang Y, Saleh M (2005) The effect of diaphyseal lengthening on the tibial growth plate. *J Bone Joint Surg.* 87-B (Suppl. III):316.

[21] Popkov D, Journeau P, Popkov A, Pedeutour B, Haumont T, Lascombes P (2012) Analysis of segmental residual growth after progressive bone lengthening in congenital lower limb deformity. *Orthop Traumatol Surg Res.*98(6):621-628.

In: Combined Stimulating Methods …
Editor: Dmitry Popkov
ISBN: 978-1-63483-028-7

Chapter V

BIOACTIVE IMPLANTS IN RECONSTRUCTIVE ORTHOPEDICS

Arnold Popkov, PhD, MD*
Scientific and Clinical Laboratory for Deformity Correction and Limb Lengthening. Federal Russian State-Financed Ilizarov Scientific Center for Restorative Traumatology and Orthopaedics, Kurgan, Russia

ABSTRACT

Detailed description of methods of external circular osteosynthesis in association with flexible intramedullary nails with bioactive coating in deformity correction are presented in Chapter V. It is concerned with surgical treatment of orthopedic disorders in such diseases as osteogenesis imperfecta. In this part of the monograph we describe various currently existing bioactive coatings of implants, used in orthopedic practice and new developing trends of this field.

Keywords: Flexible intramedullary bioactive coating, implants, intramedullary nailing

* Corresponding author: Ilizarov Scientific Center for Restorative Traumatology and Orthopaedics, 6, M.-Ulyanova Street, 640014 Kurgan, Russia; apopkov.46@mail.ru,

1. TYPES OF BIOACTIVE COATINGS AND IMPLANTS

Reconstruction of organs or skeletal parts affected by trauma or disease still remains quite challenging for the state-of-the-art traumatology and orthopedics. There are two different approaches to resolving of this problem nowadays: 1) simple substitution of an affected bone by an implant of mechanical integration or 2) creating the conditions for bone regeneration with spontaneous total recovery or by means of an implant of biological integration.

Analysis of the contemporary reference data proves that both trends are related to bioceramics. Perspectives of use of bioceramics are determined first of all by the possibility to change mechanical and biologic features of implants and their approaching to the bone tissue. We recall that the bone has complicated structure and diverse tissue constitution. Mechanical characteristics of the compact bone are determined by specific 3D position of its structural components – bone lamellae of 3-10 mkm thick [1, 2]. Bone matrix (collagen) makes up about 20-25% of total weight of bone, non-organic component (Ca phosphates) - 60-65%, content of water reaches 9-10%. Besides, there are small amounts of other organic compounds (proteins, other than collagen, polysaccharoses, lipids).

Organic bone matrix and non-organic components create a specific composition material. Contemporary bioengineering is not yet able to reproduce artificially the morphology of bone tissue in detail, thus, to achieve the same combination of biologic and mechanical features as of the bone. Nevertheless, biomaterials acting as implants should meet the following requirements:

1) Chemical features - absence of unwelcome chemical reactions with tissues and intertissue liquid, absence of corrosion;
2) Mechanical features of biomaterial should be close to those of the bone – strength (flexibility) and resistance to fatigue deformities and fractures;
3) Bioactivity of the material – absence of reaction of the immune system, osteoconductivity (ability to develop microvessels on the material surface and then ostegenic cells with formation of the bone tissue, also inside transverse pores of the optimal dimension) and osteoinductivity (ability of the material for adhesion and differentiation of mesenchymal stem cells including osteoblasts and stimulation of their osteogenic function). Osteogenity and osteoinductivity provide biointegration of implants.

Bioinert metals and alloys with ceramic coating on the bases of Ca phosphates (especially hydroxyapatite) are supposed to be the best for creating orthopedic implants for the locomotor system going through strong mechanical stresses. These materials provide biologic compatibility and significant biologic activity in bone formation around the metal.

Practical application and improvement of those implants are developed in the following directions:

1) Design of joint replacement implants: their metal load-bearing element is covered with hydroxyapatite aiming to create excessive bony sleeve providing secure contact of the metal with the bone tissue along the maximum surface, which exclude insufficient fixation of joint elements on the bone for long term.
2) Design of intramedullary implants for substitution of vast bone tissue defects resulted from trauma or radical excision in orthopedic or oncologic surgeries.
3) The reconstructive combined surgery definitely involves the second direction. As the contemporary ceramics is fragile, it covers metal layer (usually in a form of titanium, stainless steel nails of 1.5-3 mm diameter). Such covering is capable to induce reparative osteogenesis around the implant promoting bone defect substitution. Thus, a sleeve, formed along the entire implant, provides optimal conditions for healing bone fractures or pseudoarthroses, for formation of distraction regenerate in limb lengthening.

A weak point of those implants is necessity of a secondary surgery for their removal in 3-6 months after fracture consolidation, healing of bone fragments. This disadvantage is supposed to be conventional as removal of the implant is not obligatory.

Definitely, the solution of this problem suggests itself as to create an intramedullary implant made of solid composite material, which is progressively resorbed while the defect is getting filled with a newly formed bone. The first ones of those implants are composites of "hydroxyapatite – polymer" type, they manifest mechanical features similar to the bone and highly bioactive.

Development of those materials started by the end of 70s of the previous century, aiming to create artificial bone substitutes. In 1980s W. Bonfield et al. developed a composite consisted of hydroxyapatite particles and high density polyethylene [3]. Hydroxyapatite particles of 4 μm diameter were dispersed and uniformly distributed in the polymer *matrix*. Polyethylene is a typical material known for its consistency and rigidity, but manifesting no bioactivity. On the contrary, HA possesses bioactivity, but not consistency. Uniting these two materials results in products possessing consistency and bioactivity at the same time.

It was determined that if HA has a higher Young's modulus of elasticity than polyethylene, thus, this modulus of the composite "hydroxyapatite-polyethylene" rises with increase of volume ratio of HA-filler and can reach the modulus of cortical bone [3]. Nevertheless, composites lose consistency and become fragile when HA-content exceeds 45%. Y. Wang et al. also studied influence of dimension of HA-particles on mechanical properties of this composite material [4,5]. It turned out that composites with a lesser size of particles possess a higher modulus of torsion and extension and a higher tensile modulus of elasticity. The surgeon can easily pre-shape the composite during surgery, which is also an advantage of the material.

As polyethylene is not bioactive, so, when implanted, it is encapsulated with fibrous tissue and isolated from surrounding tissues. To provide bioactive properties, the content of HA particles should exceed 20% [3]. Exposure of HA-particles on the composite surface is necessary for providing bioactivity, as there should be direct contact between bioactive particles and surrounding tissues to induce the effect of osteoconductivity.

Thus, the "hydroxyapatite-polyethylene" composites with HA-content rate of 20-40% possess the consistency and Young's modulus similar to the ones of natural bone and the bioactivity. A combination of hydroxyapatite and polyethylene proposes a new material for bone substitution close to the bone by its mechanical properties. It is already used in orbital floor fractures to build up volume, and as a material for middle ear implants.

Other composites were composed of polyethylene and Bioglass® [5]. Bioglass® is bioactive glass revealing high level of bioactivity with both hard and soft tissues. In those composites the Young's modulus and microhardness grow with increase of Bioglass® content, though breaking tensile strength and strain to failure decrease. The composites build a layer of bone-like apatite on their surface [6,7].

Juhasz et al. reported about glass-ceramic A-W-polyethylene composites [8]. Glass-ceramics is distinguished for its high mechanical strength and bioactivity [7], that is why it is supposed to be an effective filler in bioactive composites. Increasing the A-W glass-ceramics content in those composites causes an increase in Young's modulus, yield strength and bending strength, and a decreased strain to failure [9]. The composites demonstrate high ability to produce apatite in simulated *interstitial fluid, also increasing with increase of* A-W glass-ceramics volume.

Composites "hydroxyapatite – poly-L-lactide" (u-HA-PLLA) contain poly-L-lactide (PLLA). This biodegradable polymer is used in fabrication of medical devices applied in clinical practice in orthopedic, cranio-maxillofacial surgery. Those devices have some weak points, like lesser strength than of the natural cortical bone, slow rate of degradation and no osteoconductivity. In order to improve bioactivity and mechanical strength of the polymer, its combination with bioactive ceramic fillers were developed. Some authors reported about composites with Ca phosphate fibers or particles of baked hydroxyapatite which are dispersed in biodegradable organic polymers. Though, those materials could not be resorbed completely. Other attempts were to add resorbable polymer to bioceramics, but those materials had low mechanical strength [10].

Shikinami et al. [11] reported development of composites "HA – PLLA", when hydroxyapatite requires no thermal processing. Unbaked powder of hydroxyapatite (u-HA) was prepared by reaction between *calcium hydrogen phosphate* anhydride ($CaHPO_4$) and calcium carbonate. It resulted in carbonate containing hydroxyapatite. HA congeries were broken and sifted to receive particles of a diameter rang 0.3-20 μm, in average - 3 μm. U-HA particles were dispersed in polymer PLLA-matrix to fabricate composites "u-HA - PLLA". The given composite possessed high mechanical strength. U-HA particles were uniformly distributed in matrix and exposed on the surface providing bioactivity. Bending strength of the material increases with increase of u-HA content. It reaches about 270 MPa with a 30 vol% u-HA filler content. This value is higher than in PLLA samples without filler and much higher than in human compound bone. Bending strength of the composite is also a little higher than in PLLA samples without u-HA and close to the value of human compound bone. Impact index of the composite with a 30 vol% u-HA filler content is much higher than the one of PLLA samples without u-HA or of human compound bone [12].

Biological properties of composites "u-HA – PLLA" were studied *in vitro* and *in vivo*. *In vitro* tests showed formation of bone-like apatite on the surface within 3 days after soaking in simulated body fluid. It suggests that the composites are bioactive. *In vivo* tests of implantation in bones of animals revealed that devices made of composites demonstrate more affinity to the bone than those made of PLLA: fibrous tissue formed on surfaces of the latter, while using of composites resulted in formation of bone-like apatite and direct contact with the bone. Histological study showed that new bone formation occurred in 2 weeks after implantation. Such bioactivity of those composites induces an early position stability of implant in bone. *Gradual degradation* of the *implanted* composite in the bone *defect* was observed to result in replacement of the *composite* by *bone* tissue. When the u-HA - PLLA composite rods were implanted in a subcutaneous layer, their bending strength preserved 85% of the initial value in 8 weeks and 80% in 25 weeks, while the molecular weight of the rods reduced to 20% of the initial value over the same period [13,14].

Healing of a fractured human bone normally requires over 8-12 weeks, though the healing period is determined by various parameters, like fracture location, stability of bone fragments, patient's age. Stability of osteosynthesis is believed to be a very important factor during healing, so, in order to maintain stable fixation during this period, the mechanical strength of an intramedullary or on-bone device should be preserved. Despite the fact that the u-HA – PLLA composite demonstrated a faster degradation in bone defects than PLLA alone, fabricated with the same technique, but devices made of this composite preserve mechanical firmness during the entire period of fracture healing.

Shukinami et al. reported total degradation of rods for bone fixation made of "u-HA – PLLA" composite in approximately 4.5-5 years after being implanted: passages created in the distal femoral condylar for implanting were almost totally filled in with new bone [11]. There was no inflammatory response to biodegradation or bone defect substitution.

Thus, analysis of literature revealed that research in ceramics-polymer composites creation reached the level of commercially affordable proposals and the concept of combining of non-organic and organic components seems to be logic in developing material for bone reconstruction.

Choice of this or that material depends on medical-biologic characteristics of the bone defect as well as on a concrete clinical case. So, solution of this problem is possible upon availability of the whole range of biomaterials. Choosing the most appropriate material for the concrete case allows to the surgeon to shift from reconstructive-substitutive principle of treatment to a higher level of bioengineering.

Currently, tissue engineering is one of the youngest branches of medicine, it is based on the principles of molecular biology and genetic engineering. A multidisciplinary approach used in this sphere is aimed to create new biocomposite materials for recovery of lost functions of certain tissues or organs [15,16].

Basic principles of this approach are development and implantation of bases made of biodegradable material into the damaged organ or tissue, which are used in association with donor cells and/or bioactive materials. In the latest years, new technologies allow to extract bone morphogenic proteins (BMPs/BMP-2 and BMP-7) and use them in clinical practice.

Recombinant human osteogenic Protein-1 (rhOP-1), inducing *in vivo* formation of new bone tissue and possessing specific activity similar to natural osteogenic protein, stimulates proliferation and differentiation of osteoblasts *in vitro*. It is able to induce formation of bone tissue by stimulation of mesenchymal stem cells and their following differentiation into precursor osteogenic cells. Administration of rhOP-1 into the bone defect gap and fracture site provides total recovery of the bone in 30 months.

One of the major tasks of tissue engineering in treatment of bone pathologies is creation of synthetic composites which are able in combination with bioactive molecules to induce osteogenesis as well as chondrogenesis in reconstruction of joint surfaces (the latter has not found a practical application yet). Besides, such materials should possess certain properties of the bone [17,18,19]:

- to scaffold the defect volume,
- to possess osteoinductive capacity,
- to be biocompatible, i.e. to be able to biodegrade and not to provoke inflammatory response of the recipient.

All those properties together allow to such materials along with a supportive function to provide biointegration – ingrowth of cells and vessels into the implant structure, and stimulate bone tissue formation around the implant.

Tissue engineering implies using of cells in complex with biologic or artificial matrixes which conduct cells in the process of reparation. Implant fabrication should be rather cheap and clinical application with osteoinductive capacities should guarantee consolidation of injured bone in the shortest period possible: consolidation of a simple fracture of long bones should not exceed 3-4 weeks, as for formation of the distraction regeneration in bone lengthening, the time of regenerate mineralization allowing to remove the external fixator should tend to zero (the process of mineralization must coincide with the process of formation of organic matrix).

Currently, the intramedullary implant in a shape of a titanium HA-coated wire meets all the requirements: production is rather cheap, practical application does not require use of expensive donor cells and artificial bioactive materials (OP-1, rhOP-1). Intramedullary space, bone marrow and endostium contain the entire set of morphogenetic proteins, ferments and growth factors, a great number of mesenchymal stem cells and endosteal osteogenic cells, needed for differentiation to osteoblasts and proliferation of the bone substance around the intramedullary nails.

Concept of Bone Tissue Formation on the Intramedullary Implant Surface

Nowadays, understanding of basics of the reparative regeneration in "skeletal tissues" provides development of tissue engineering in orthopedics and traumatology, first of all because of unsatisfactory time and results of fracture healing. When the contemporary science states that fractures require at least 12 weeks for healing and real time of patient's rehabilitation takes 10-12 months, when the healing index in limb lengthening 45 days/cm [20-22], the situation naturally needs development of medical technologies stimulating the reparative process.

The Ilizarov scientific school always held to the concept of sufficiency of proper body reserve for healing of limb fractures and maintenance of optimal conditions for reparative bone regeneration that means:

- thorough, preferably close reduction of bone fragments,
- stable fixation of bone fragments,
- low invasive surgery,
- adequate blood supply of the fracture or limb lengthening site,
- optimal rate and rhythm of distraction,
- functional weight bearing of the limb during treatment.

Economic expediency is the basis of elaboration of the method of transosseous osteosynthesis aimed to osteogenetic induction. In 2001 D. Popkov suggested to lengthen long tubular bones by means of flexible intramedullary nailing. First, Ilizarov Scientific Center (Kurgan, Russia) started to apply the technique, then Pediatric Orthopedic Center (Nancy, France). As a result, reinforcement of reparative osteogenesis around flexible nails and reduction of healing time were noted [23-25].

In our opinion, the intramedullary osteosynthesis by nails with bioactive coating performs two functions – provides additional stability of bone fragments as well as all osteoconductive and osteoinductive conditions for reparative bone tissue regeneration characteristic to HA-based materials.

From the economic point of view, the production technology of nails with bioactive calcium phosphate coating is an inexpensive process [26,27], and intramedullary positioning of the implant excludes necessity of additional cultivation of high-cost growth and cell factors.

Titanium nails are coated with biologic or synthetic hydroxyapatite produced by low temperature method [28]. According to the results of electronic microscopy, the present HA sample is a powder mixture with pallets inclusions of nanoscale structure of 10-100 nm diameter. According to X-ray phase analysis, the powder is a heterogeneous hydroxyapatite mixture of hexagonal and monoclinal structure with the internal surface area over 70 m^2/g. The coating technology of titanium nails of 1.8mm diameter is based on electrochemical deposition. In average the coating thickness is 85±3.0 μm, surface roughness – 5.5±0.01 μm. According to the results of AFM of fine resolution, the coating pattern consists of nodules of approximately 100 nm diameter, of approximately 35 nm height, and flaky fragments. They form spherulites of about 5 μm in diameter and up to 300 nm in height. In the middle of spherulites and in between them there are transverse pores of the diameter below 1-2 μm reaching metal base surface. Electronographic image of titanium coating of nails viewed micropore diameter of 2 to 5 μm (figure 29).

The flexible intramedullary nailing with bioactive HA-coating allows to influence on the bone marrow activity stimulating endosteal bone formation by the very presence of the nail. Its internal stress induces the function of mesenchymal tissue of the bone marrow (mechanoinduction of osteogenesis). This method of osteoinduction is characterized by low traumatism, it preserves the nutrient artery, and excludes possibility of delayed consolidation.

Formation of bone tissue on the ceramic implant surface requires adhesion of certain molecules. The bone structure is hierarchically organized in various ranges of length – from macro- to nanoscale, thus, the implant structure also should be hierarchically organized in three levels: macro- , micro- and nano-. Besides, nano surface pattern should be approximately 100 nm in order to conform with cell receptors and the pores are needed of micro- and macro dimensions. The recommended dimension of micro pores is at least 300 μm which provides nutrition and cell distribution on the implant surface as well as formation of capillaries in it.

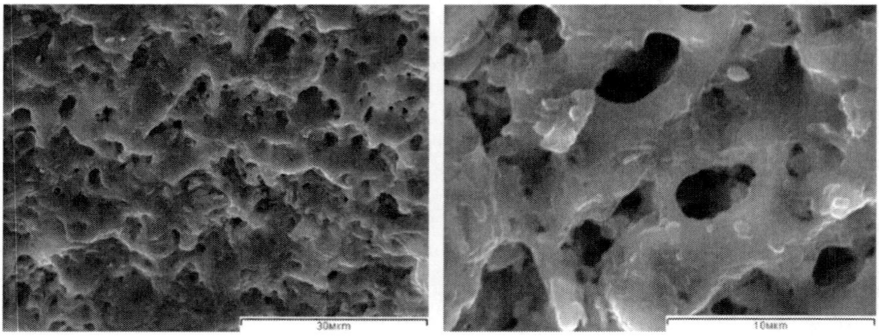

(a) (b)

Figure 29. Surface of the intramedullary titanium nail (scanning electron microscope) x1500 (a); x5000 (b).

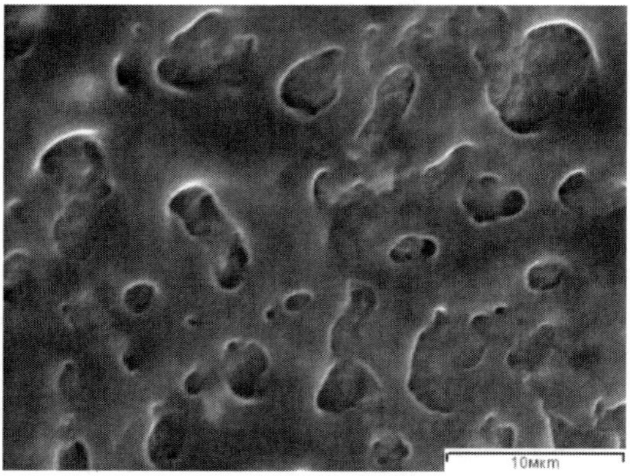

Figure 30. Surface of an intramedullary nail at 26th day of experimental study (scanning electron microscope, x3000). Through holes in the protein film can be seen the hydroxyapatite coating.

Studies of ectopic osteogenesis on the ceramic implant surface showed that bone tissue formation is obligatory preceded by cell migration and angiogenesis which are observed only if there is a sufficient amount of micropores, otherwise, ectopic formation of the new bone can slow down or fail. It is well known that not porous materials don't manifest osteoinductive properties.

We determined that immediately after implantation of biomaterial, proteins of blood and extracellular matrix (figure 30) – fibronectin, osteocalcin, bone sialoproteins, immunoglobulin, albumin, etc. – are absorbed on the biomaterial surface.

We believe that osteoinduction is related both to the design of the implant surface pattern and to a biological phenomenon of inflammatory response developing after implanting of biomaterials [29,30]. Caplan A.I. and Boyan B.D. [31] hypothesized that initial inflammatory response to implanting of biomaterials stimulated factors attracting mesenchymal stem cells. One of them can be prostaglandin E2 (PGE2) produced by macrophages accumulated around biomaterials during the inflammatory phase [32,33]. The microrough surface, unique for osteoinductive materials, reported to stimulate production of PGE2 by macrophages [32] and PGE2 possesses hemotoxic features towards human mesenchymal stem cells and stimulates their osteogenic differentiation.

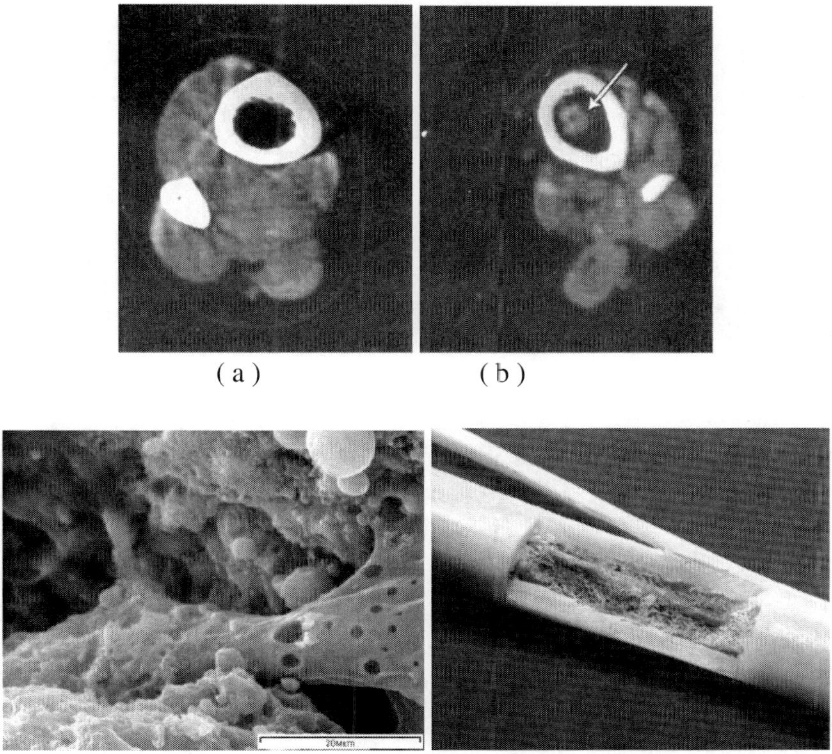

(a) (b) (c) (d)

Figure 31. The bone tissue formation around intramedullary nail: intact tibia, computed tomography (a); lengthened tibia, after nail removal (b); bone trabeculae formation on the HA-coated surface of intramedullary nail (c); cancellous bone tissue filled in the space around the intramedullary nail (d).

As a result of flexible intramedullary nailing, a certain bony sleeve forms around the nail because of inducing of the local osteogenesis. Figure 31 demonstrates CT images of dog's tibiae – intact and undergone intramedullary osteosynthesis. Shades of bony sleeve around the canal of intramedullary nail are clearly seen inside the marrow cavity. Thickness of a mineralized wall of this "sleeve" ranges from 1 to 3 mm. The bone tissue ingrows into pores of the implant surface and rapidly fills in all the space of marrow cavity firmly uniting nails with endosteum (figure31). Cancellous bone forms as a natural bone scaffold in fracture.

Osteoconductive and osteoinductive properties of flexible implants, that we developed, provide directional growth of new bone tissue in the fracture site, as well as in the limb lengthening gap, in correction of systemic diseases (osteogenesis imperfecta, Ollier disease, fibrous osteodysplasia, rickets-like diseases), in substitution of bone cysts; they also favor finishing of bone histogenesis in postnatal period in place of cartilaginous or connective matrix [34].

REFERENCES

[1] Ripamonti U, Crooks J, Khoali L, Roden L (2009) The induction of bone formation by coral-derived calcium carbonate/hydroxyapatite constructs *Biomaterials.* 30(7):1428–1439.

[2] Rivera EM, Araiza M, Brostow W et al. (1999) Synthesis of hydroxyapatite from eggshells. *Matter Lett.* 41:128-134.

[3] Bonfield W, Wang. M, Tanner KE (1998) Interfaces in analogue biomaterials. *Acta Mater.* 46(7):2509–2518.

[4] Wang J, Layrolle P, Stigter M, de Groot K (2004) Biomimetic and electrolytic calcium phosphate coatings on titanium alloy: physicochemical characteristics and cell attachment. *Biomaterials.* 25:583–592.

[5] Wang Y, Khor KA, Cheang P (1998) Thermal Spraying of Functionally Graded Calcium Phosphate Coatings for Biomedical Implants. *J. Therm. Spray Technol.* 3:50–57.

[6] Kokubo T, Kushitani H, Sakka S et al. (1990) Solutions able to reproduce in vivo surface-structure changes in bioactive glass-ceramic A-W. *J. Biomed. Mater Res.* 24:721–734.

[7] Kokubo T, Takadama H (2006) How useful is SBF in predicting in vivo bone bioactivity? *Biomaterials.* 27:2907–2915.

[8] Juhasz JA, Best SM, Bonfield W, Kawashita M, Miyata N, Kokubo T, Nakamura T (2003) Apatite-forming ability of glass-ceramic apatite-wollastonite - polyethylene composites: effect of filler content. *J. Mater Sci. Mater Med.* 14(6):489-495.

[9] Juhasz JA, Best SM, Brooks R, Kawashita M, Miyata N, Kokubo T, Nakamura T, Bonfield W (2004) Mechanical properties of glass-ceramic A-W-polyethylene composites: effect of filler content and particle size. *Biomaterials.* 25(6):949-955.

[10] Verheyen CC, de Wijn JR, van Blitterswijk CA, de Groot K (1992) Evaluation of hydroxylapatite/poly (L-lactide) composites: mechanical behavior. *J. Biomed. Mater Res.* 26(10):1277-1296.

[11] Shikinami Y, Matsusue Y, Nakamura T (2005) The complete process of bioresorption and bone replacement using devices made of forged composites of raw hydroxyapatite particles/poly l-lactide (F-u-HA/PLLA). *Biomaterials.* 26:5542-5551.

[12] Shikinami Y, Okuno M (1999) Bioresorbable devices made of forged composites of hydroxyapatite (HA) particles and poly-L-lactide (PLLA): Part I. Basic Characteristics. *Biomaterials.* 20(9):859-877.

[13] Furukawa T, Matsusue Y, Yasunaga T, Nakagawa Y, Shikinami Y, Okuno M, Nakamura T (2000) Bone bonding ability of a new biodegradable composite for internal fixation of bone fractures. *Clin. Orthop. Relat. Res.* 379:247-258.

[14] Furukawa T, Matsusue Y, Yasunaga T, Shikinami Y, Okuno M, Nakamura T (2000) Biodegradation behavior of ultra-high-strength hydroxyapatite/poly (L-lactide) composite rods for internal fixation of bone fractures. *Biomaterials.* 21(9):889-898.

[15] Langer R, Vacanti JP (1993) Tissue engineering. *Science.* 260:920–926.

[16] Spector M (1999) Basis Principles of Tissue Engineering in Tissue Engineering Application in Maxillofacial Surgery and Periodontics. Ed. S. Lynch; Quintessence Publishing Co. Inc: pp3–17.

[17] Yannas IV, Hansbrough J, Ehrlich N (1984) What criteria should be used for designing artificial skin replacements and how well do the current grafting materials meet these criteria? *J. Trauma.* 24:29.

[18] Reddi AH, Weintroub S, Muthukumaran N (1987) Biological principles of bone induction. Orthop Clin N Amer. 18:207–212.

[19] Reddi AH (1998) Role of morphogenetic proteins in skeletal tissue engineering and regeneration. *Nat. Biotechnol.* 16(3) :247–252.

[20] Caton J (1994) Comment établir un plan d'égalisation? Eléments du choix. In: Les inégalités de longueur des membres: sous la direction de A. Diméglio et al; Paris–Milan–Barcelone: MASSON. pp174–176.

[21] Glorion Ch (2000) Complications des allongements des membres. Cahiers d'enseignement de la SOFCOT; Elsevier. pp165–182.

[22] Launay F, Jouve JL, Guillaume E et al. (2001) Les allongementsprogressifs de l'avant-bras chez l'enfant. A propos d'une série de 14 cas. *Rev. Chir. Orthop.* 87:786–795.

[23] Popkov D, Popkov A, Haumont T, Journeau P, Lascombes P (2010) Flexible intramedullary nail use in limb lengthening. *J. Pediatr Orthop.* 30:910-918.

[24] Popkov D, Journeau P, Popkov A, Haumont T, Lascombes P (2010) Ollier's disease limb lenghtening: Should intramedullary nailing be combined with circular external fixation? *Orthop. Traumatol. Surg. Res.* 96:348-353.

[25] Popkov D, Lascombes P, Popkov A, Journeau P, Haumont T (2012) Role of the flexible intramedullary nailing in limb lengthening in children: comparative study based on the series of 295 lengthenins. *European Orthopaedics Traumatology*. 3:17-24.

[26] Guseev VV, Tretiakova EM, Ivanova LR (2000) Ceramic materials reinforced with phosphate binders [in russian]. *Glass and ceramics.* 3:36–38.

[27] Guseeva TI, Guseev VV, Leonova LA (2009) Preparation of hydroxyapatite powder in the liquid-phase synthesis [in russian]. *News of Tomsk polytechnic university*. 315(3):47-50.

[28] Talashova IA, Silantieva TA (2007) The laboratory excretion of calcium phosphate compounds from the bone tissue of cattle and the determination of their composition by the method of electrone-probe microanalysis [in russian]. *Genij ortopedii*. 4:71–75.

[29] Popkov AV, Osipenko AV (2008) Tissue regeneration in limb lengthening [in russian]. Moscow, GEOTAR-Media. 239p.

[30] Le Nihouannen D, Daculsi G, Saffarzadeh A et al. (2005) Ectopic bone formation by microporous calcium phosphate ceramic particles in sheep muscles. *Bone.* 36:1086–1093.

[31] Caplan AI, Boyan BD (1994) Endochondral Bone Formation: The Lineage Cascade. *Bone.* 8(1):1–46.

[32] Thomsen P, Gretzer C (2001) Macrophage interactions with modified material surfaces. *Curr. Opin Solid State a Mater Sci.* 5(2–3):163–176.

[33] Refai AK, Textor M, Brunette DM, Waterfield JD (2004) Effect of titanium surface topography on macrophage activation and secretion of proinflamatory cytokines and chemokines. *J. Biomed. Mater Res. A.* 70:194–205.

[34] Popkov A, Popkov D (2012) Bioactif Implants in Traumatology and Orthopaedics [in russian]. Irkutsk, Russia: NSRS SO RAMN, 438p.

2. Use of Intramedullary Bioactive Nailing in Osteogenesis Imperfecta

Deformity Correction and Intramedullary Telescopic Constructions

Basic surgical methods of treatment of deformities in children affected with osteogenesis imperfecta are corrective osteotomies and a basic mode of osteosynthesis is intramedullary [1-7,11,17,18,20]. Considering the fact that in OI all the limbs are involved, it is recommended to use reference data for treatment planning [7,8,15]. When levels and amount of deformity correction are determined, a number of required osteotomies and amount of correction at each level is calculated [10,13]. It is important to correct all the deformity components of the entire limb within one surgical session, as the deformities are often counter-directed and compensate the above and below segment axis [6,10,20]. Preventive osteosynthesis of long bones as well as osteosynthesis in fractures are performed using intramedullary telescopic transphyseal constructions [3,12,17,19,20].

Among the basic intramedullary telescopic constructions there are

1. Flexible intramedullary nailing (FIN) [4,10];
2. Telescopic Bailey-Dubow nail [1-3];
3. Telescopic Fassier-Duval nail [7,14,20].

But the use of those telescopic systems is not devoid of complications [9,21].

We have developed and use transphyseal osteosynthesis with HA-coated bioactive intramedullary nails. Specific features of the coating providing osteoconductive and osteoinductive characteristics [14,16] are described in the previous chapter.

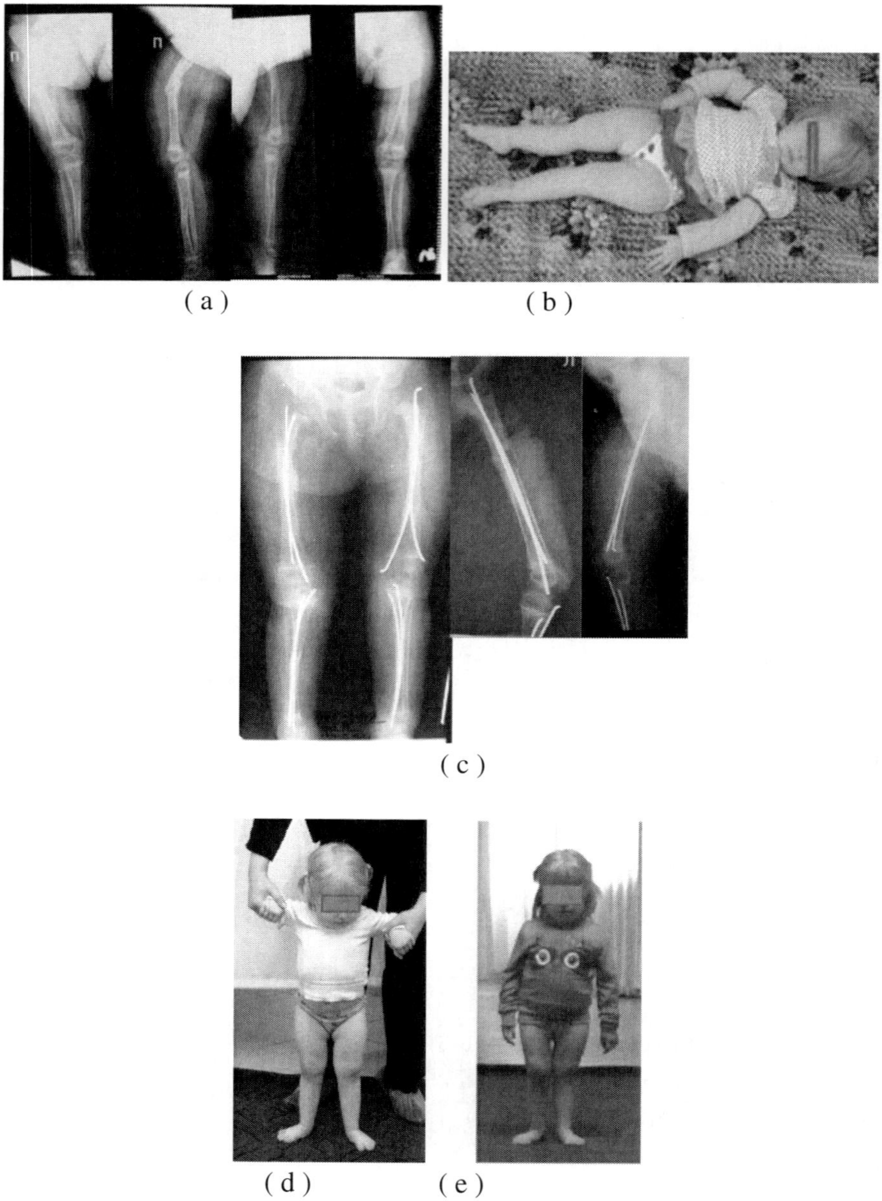

Figure 32. Application example of intramedullary transphyseal flexible osteosynthesis in a two-year-old female patient: X-rays of right and left lower limbs before treatment (a), photo of the patient (b); before surgery the child could not walk and stand. AP X-rays of limbs, lateral X-rays of femurs after insertion of flexible nails (c), the child began to stand with weight bearing on limbs in 3 months (d) and to walk independently in 5 months (e).

The procedure (figure 32) starts with insertion of elastic, pre-curved along the entire length, mostly titanium nails of 1.5 to 4 mm diameter. The nails are smoothly contoured that produces two opposing curves. They are inserted towards each other from the opposite epiphyses or apophyses transphyseally. An important aspect of the passage through the physis is use of a trocar or a surgical awl and performance of this maneuver at a single-attempt in order to avoid excessive trauma of the growth zone.

The nails can be advanced through the medullary canal to the opposite epiphysis without prior reaming. If the canal is very narrow or absent at all, the reaming of these parts of the bone is performed through the same approaches as osteotomies. Very often realignment osteotomies require one or several incisions to advance the wire under visual control.

FIN is the most effective method of osteosynthesis in deformity correction of the upper limbs. Indications for the surgical treatment are more frequent in forearm deformities, impairing use of the upper extremity in daily routine [6,19]. It is the small diameter of forearm bones that implies application of intramedullary nails of the 1.5-3 mm diameter for osteosynthesis of bone fragments after corrective osteotomies (figure 33).

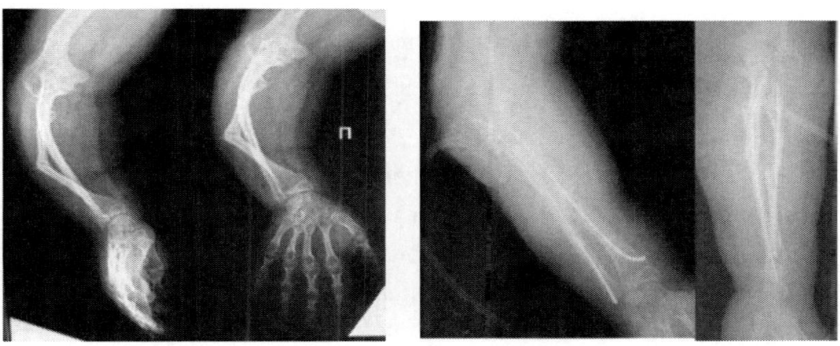

(a) (b)

Figure 33. Example of forearm deformity correction: X-rays of the forearm before surgery (a), after deformity correction and intramedullary flexible nailing (b).

Strong and Weak Points of This Method of Osteosynthesis

HA-coated FIN definitely preserves all advantages of the intramedullary elastic osteosynthesis with titanium or steel nails [4,10]. This method of osteosynthesis can be used almost in all bone dimensions. Besides, if the marrow cavity is obliterated, preliminary reaming of fragments, even moderate, allows to insert elastic nails of a small diameter. This method of osteosynthesis permits to stabilize bone fragments in multilevel osteotomies.

Elasticity of osteosynthesis provides distribution of the weight bearing along the entire medullar canal which is favorable for bone consolidation and does not impair strength properties of cortical plates. Intramedullary telescopic constructions prevent secondary fractures, even if they occur, bone fragments remain stable without significant displacement. Also, telescopic character of FIN scaffolds the bone while it is growing; stabilizing features of intramedullary nails are preserved if they overlap each other by 30% of their proper length and more. Besides, the HA-coating dramatically decreases nail migration in the long-term follow-up.

Results of assessment of how hydroxyapatite coating influences on preservation of mineral density in the operated segment are presented below.

A disadvantage of the technique is exclusion and then restriction within several weeks of the total weight bearing on the operated limb. Such a motion behavior causes decrease of the bone mineral density. In the long-term follow-up it is necessary to change nails while the bone growing in length and in diameter.

Combined Technique

In the Ilizarov Center we use combined osteosynthesis (external fixation and flexible intramedullary nailing) for severe multilevel deformities [14].

The technique is supposed for correction of deformities of lower limbs in children affected with osteogenesis imperfecta. It is based on a combined application of the transosseous osteosynthesis with the Ilizarov device and intramedullary osteosynthesis with bioactive HA-coated nails which provide prophylactics of deformity relapse. Application of the Ilizarov fixator allows to start weight-bearing on the operated limb from first post-operative days and to prevent secondary torsion deformities.

Technical Performance in Limb Deformities

Taking into consideration that lower limb deformities involve, as a rule, both the femur and tibia, polysegmental osteosynthesis of the limb is recommended, i.e. both segments should be operated simultaneously. Surgical procedure can be monofocal or bifocal in each segment depending on extensivity and amount of the deformity (figure 34).

The surgery begins with insertion of intramedullary titanium nails with bioactive coating. In order to perform it, an oblique tunnel is made through a cortical layer into medullary cavity via a cutaneous incision of 8-10 mm long on lateral and medial surfaces of the metaphysis by means of a 4-5 mm diameter awl. An HA-coated nail is inserted through the tunnel. The nail diameter (2-3.5 mm) depends on the diameter of the intramedullary canal. In this pathology the marrow canal is often irregular or even absent at some locations, thus, insertion of nails is challenging for a surgeon and requires specific instruments.

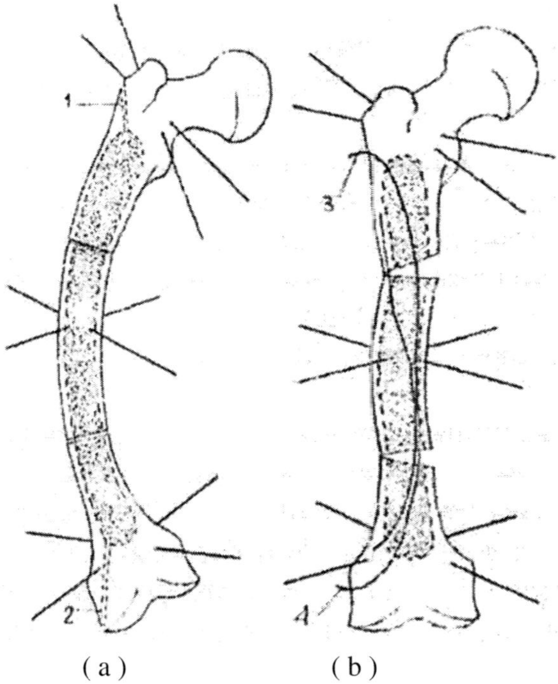

Figure 34. Bone segment scheme of application of intramedullary nails in the combines technique: the segment before deformity correction (a), 1 and 2 - canals for intramedullary nail insertion; the segment after deformity correction and intramedullary nail insertion (b), 3 and 4 - inserted intramedullary nails into the medullary cavity.

A special device (figure 35) can be used to guide and ensure a necessary direction for insertion of the nail according to the shape of medullary canal and bone deformity. It is also important, if the medullary cavity is absent (eburnation) or of a small diameter and needed to be drilled with a wire.

A flexible curved nail is inserted in the medullary cavity via guide. If the medullary cavity is patent, the nail is usually easy to introduce manually up to the opposite metaphysis. When the guide is taken out, a free nail end is cut and bent. A U-shaped bend should prevent nail migration into the medullary cavity during distraction, and, at the same time, make it possible to grip the tip with a special instrument for removal in several months after limb lengthening.

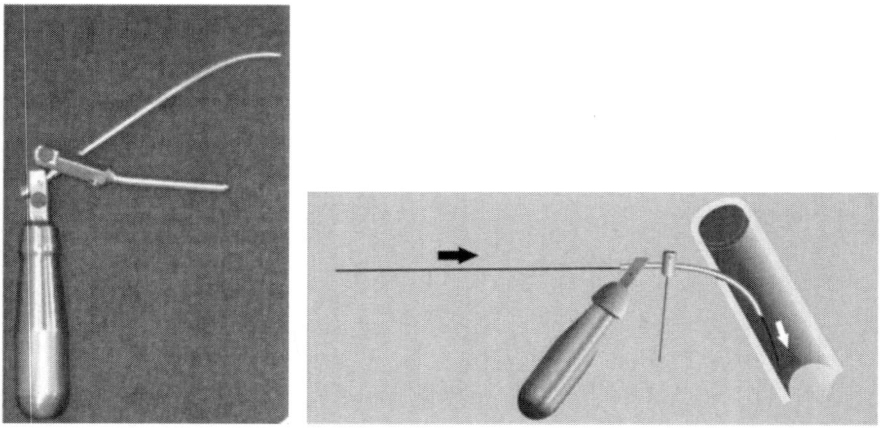

(a) (b)

Figure 35. Tubular guide for intramedullary nails: photo (a), scheme of positioning in bone (b), the nail in the canal.

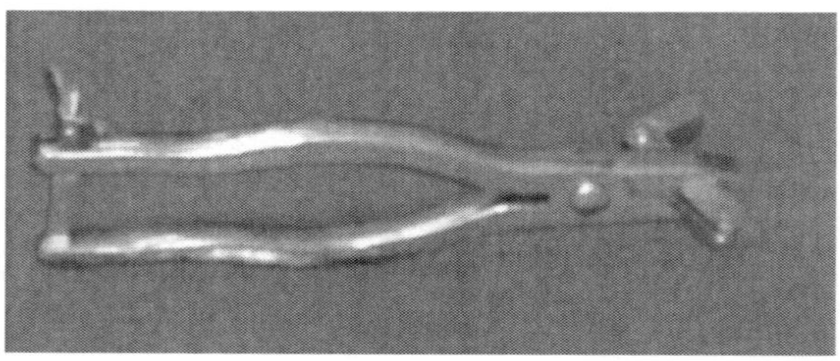

(a)

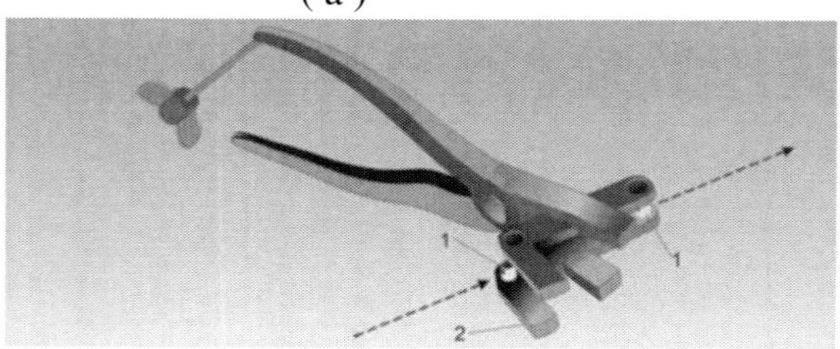

(b)

Figure 36. Special pusher for longitudinal nail insertion: photo (a), scheme (b), 1 - guides, 2 - hammer spot.

If there are small thin bone trabeculae crossing the medullary cavity and the surgeon does not intend to traumatize the canal by drilling, a special pusher (figure 36) is used.

A severe bone deformity associated with osteoporosis usually renders impossible to insert the nail by the full length of the medullary canal at one time (as the nail easily perforates the bone cortex), so at the level of deformity apex (if angulation is up to 20°) a corrective hinge osteotomy should be performed. Then, having performed an acute axial alignment of the limb, the nail is introduced in the proximal bone fragment. If the deformity exceeds 20°, the intramedullary nailing is technically feasible only after closing wedge osteotomy at the deformity apex and its acute correction.

When the nails are inserted, then the soft tissues are sutured and transosseous osteosynthesis of a shorten limb segment is performed with Ilizarov fixator assembled according to the goals of the surgeon. A clinical case illustrating this surgical technique is presented below.

A Clinical Case

A female patient K., 6 years old. Diagnosis: osteogenesis imperfecta, combined deformities of lower limbs and contractures of hip and knee joints (figure 37 a,b). In anamnesis: multiple close fractures of lower limb bones treated conservatively.

The patient underwent a consecutive deformity correction of lower limbs and flexible intramedullary nailing with HA-coating (figure 37 c,d). Rehabilitation took an average recovery time, control of long-term follow-up revealed complete functional recovery of the limbs and no deformity relapse in 18 months after treatment (figure 37e).

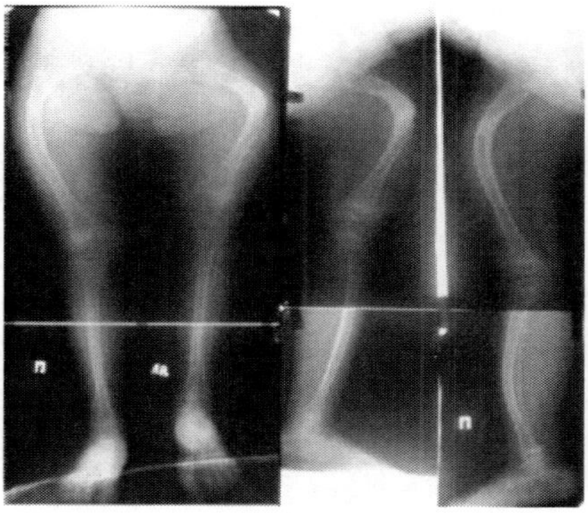

(a)

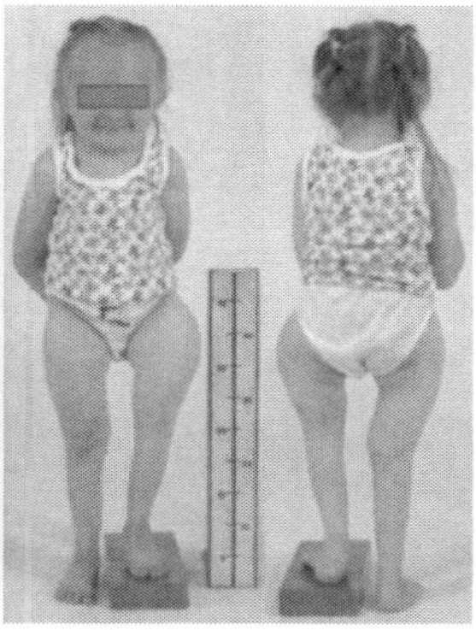

(b)

Figure 37. (Continued).

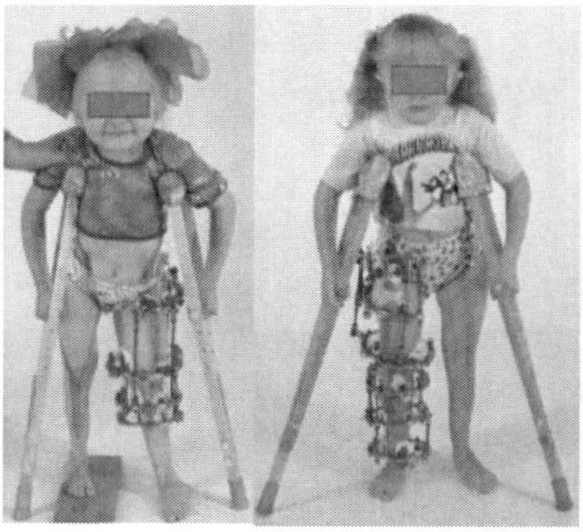

(c)

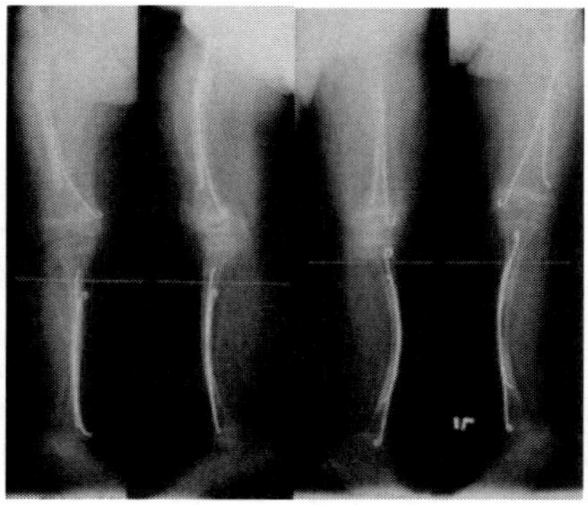

(d)

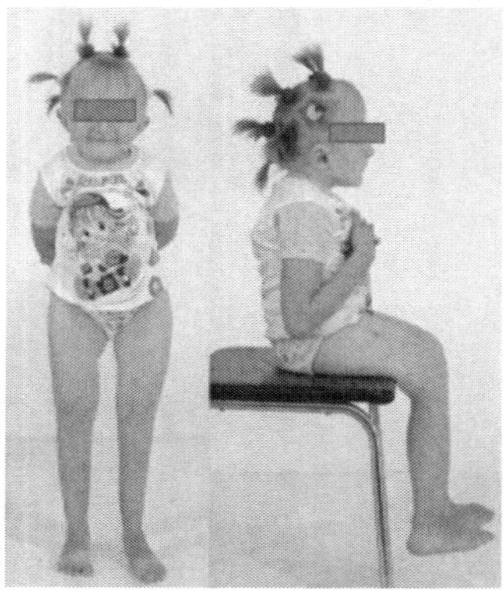

(e)

Figure 37. Female patient K., 6 years old, osteogenesis imperfecta: X-rays of lower limbs before treatment (a), photo before treatment (b), photo during deformity correction with Ilizarov device (c), X-rays of lower limbs after treatment (d), photo and functional abilities of lower limbs in one year after treatment (e).

Bone Mineral Density Study Results

In twenty patients of the age range from 4 to 27, who underwent polysegmental combined osteosynthesis with the Ilizarov frame and HA-coated flexible intramedullary nailing, bone mineral density was assessed (dual-photon bone densitometer “GE Lunar Corp”, USA) at the metaphyseal level of operated segments. Also measurements were taken at L2, L3, L4 levels. Assessments were done in 30 and 60 days after surgery, in 6 and 12 months after removal of the Ilizarov device.

The aim of study was to evaluate dynamics of bone mineral density of operated segments and lumbar vertebrae in conditions of an early activation of patients in postoperative period and using bioactive implants. It is worth of mentioning, that during the study period the patients were not administrated bisphosphonates.

Before surgery the bone mineral density value was 53.6% ($p<0.001$) of the value of healthy people in a proximal femoral metaphysis, where nail insertion was planned (table V.2.1). By the 30th postoperative day the bone mineral density increased by 9.6% ($p<0.05$) of the initial one. By the time of Ilizarov frame removal (60 days) it reached 19.5% ($p<0.001$). In 6 and 12 months the bone mineral density value always remained higher then initial.

Such a bone mineral density dynamics is noted in a distal femoral metaphysis (table V.2.2), a proximal tibial metaphysis (table V.2.3).

Table V.2.1. Mineral density in a proximal femoral metaphysis (*M*±*SD*)

Period	Mineral density, g/cm^2	
	Metaphysis	Cortices
Normal value	1.570±0.108	1.680±0.101
Before surgery	0.841±0.059	1.277±0.102
After surgery		
D 30	0.922±0.054*	1.433±0.086*
D 60	1.005±0.080*	1.519±0.106*
After frame removal		
6 months	1.051±0.079*	1.289±0.104*
12 months	1.062±0.069*	1.340±0.094*

Note: * significant difference ($p<0.05$, Student's t-test) in comparison to the initial value.

Table V.2.2. Mineral density in a distal femoral metaphysis (*M*±*SD*)

Period	Mineral density, g/cm^2	
	Metaphysis	Cortices
Normal value	1.410±0.098	1.546±0.106
Before surgery	0.635±0.051	0.983±0.079
After surgery		
D 30	0.710± 0.046*	1.079±0.086*
D 60	0.786± 0.044*	1.167±0.070*
After frame removal		
6 months	0.785±0.058*	1.168±0.064*
12 months	0.797±0.048*	1.174±0.094*

Note: * significant difference ($p<0.05$, Student's t-test) in comparison to the initial value.

Table V.2.3. Mineral density in a proximal tibial metaphysis (*M*±*SD*)

Period	Mineral density, g/cm^2	
	Metaphysis	Cortices
Normal value	1.571±0.094	1.736±0,127
Before surgery	0.705±0.049	1.043±0,073
After surgery		
D 30	0.854±0.068*	1.172±0.082*
D 60	0.874±0.070*	1.211±0.073*
After frame removal		
6 months	0.885±0.071*	1.218±0.085*
12 months	0.890±0.053*	1.215±0.079*

Note: * significant difference ($p<0.05$, Student's t-test) in comparison to the initial value.

Table V.2.4. Amount of mineral substances in L2, L3, L4 vertebrae (*M*±*SD*)

Period	Amount of mineral substances; g
Normal value	59.10 ± 4.10
Before surgery	47.30 ± 2.84
After surgery	
D 30	49.10 ± 2.71
D 60	53.0 ± 2.82*
After frame removal	
6 months	54.60 ± 2.64*
12 months	54.80 ± 3.12*

Note: * significant difference ($p<0.05$, Student's t-test) in comparison to the initial value.

Total amount of mineral substance in L2, L3, L4 vertebrae (table V.2.4) in patients before treatment was in average by 20% less than in healthy people. By the 30th postoperative day there was a tendency to bone mineral density increase, in average by 3.8% ($p<0.05$). In 60 days after surgery the increase reached 12.1% and became statistically significant in comparison to the preoperative bone mineral density level ($p<0.05$). Ilizarov frame removal did not influence on mineral substance content in the spine. During the following year of follow-up its amount did not change.

Conclusion

Thus, we can remark, that combined techniques of osteosynthesis with application of bioactive implants used in patients with osteogenesis imperfecta for limb deformity correction enable to achieve a secure orthopedic outcome: correction of both angular and torsion deformities in femur and tibia simultaneously. Duration of external fixation does not exceed 1.5-2 months. Combined osteosynthesis used at the beginning of treatment in deformity correction becomes the intramedullary one after removal of the external fixator and prevents deformity relapse.

Combined osteosynthesis allowing to weight-bearing on the operated limb and mobilization of patients from first postoperative days allows to preserve and even to increase bone mineral density. First, this effect results from an early verticalization of patients and correspondingly an early weight-bearing on operated limbs. The second important element is HA-coated intramedullary nailing. Hypothetically, applying it, we can suggest an effect of decreasing or even excluding of mobilization of skeleton calcium repository (of intact and operated bones). The third factor is biointegration of implants [14,16]. It provides an increased stability of osteosynthesis of bone fragments, which advances bone consolidation and frame removal. All together these factors promote motion activity of a patient, necessary for preserving skeletal mineral density.

References

[1] Bailey Cole WG (1993) Early surgical management of severe forms of osteogenesis imperfecta. *Am. J. Med. Genet.* 45:270–274.

[2] Bailey RW, Dubow HI (1981) Evolution of the concept of an extensible wire accomodating to normal longitudinal bone growth: clinical considerations and implications. *Clin. Orthop.* 159:157–170.

[3] Bilsel N, Beyzadeoglu T, Kafadar A (2000) Application of Bailey–Dubow rods in the treatment of Osteogenesis Imperfecta. *Eur. J. Orthop. Surg. Traumatol.* 10:183–187.

[4] Boutaud B, Laville JM (2004) L'embrochage centromédullaire coulissant dans l'ostéogenèse imparfaite. *Rev. Chir. Orthop.* 90:304–311.

[5] Cole WG. Early surgical management of severe forms of osteogenesis imperfect (1993) *Am. J. Med. Genet.* 45:270–274.

[6] Esposito P, Plotkin H (2008) Surgical treatment of osteogenesis imperfecta: current concepts. *Curr. Opin. Pediatr*. 20:52–57.

[7] Fassier F, Glorieux F (1999) Osteogeneis imperfecta in the child. Cahiers d'enseignement de la SOFCOT. Paris:Expansion Scientifique Française. pp235–252.

[8] Glorieux FH. Osteogenesis imperfecta (2008) *Best Pract. Res. Clin. Rheumatol.* 22:85–100.

[9] Larson T, Brighton B, Esposito P et al. (2010) High reoperation rate and failed expansion in lower extremity expandable rods in osteogenesis imperfecta. In: Proceedings of the Annual Meeting of the Pediatric Orthopaedic Society of North America (POSNA), Waikoloa, Hawaii.

[10] Lascombes P (2010) Flexible intramedullary nailing. Springer-Verlag Berlin Heidelberg.

[11] McHale KA, Tenuata TJ, Tosi LL, McKay DW (1994) Percutaneous intramedullary fixation of long bone deformity in severe osteogenesis imperfecta. *Clin. Orthop*. 305:242–248.

[12] Popkov DA, Kononovich NA, Shutov RB (2014) The effect of tibial transphyseal reinforcement on the growth and leg tissues. *Russian Journal of Physiology*. 100(7):81-90.

[13] Popkov D, Lascombes P, Berte N, Hetzel L, Ribeiro Baptista B, Popkov A, Journeau P (2014) The normal radiological anteroposterior alignment of the lower limb in children. *Skeletal Radiol*. DOI: 10.1007/s00256-014-1953-z.

[14] Popkov A, Popkov D (2012) Bioactif Implants in Traumatology and Orthopaedics [in russian]. Irkutsk, Russia: NSRS SO RAMN.

[15] Rauch F, Glorieux FH (2004) Osteogenesis imperfecta. *Lancet.* 363:1377–1385.

[16] Ripamonti U (2000) Smart biomaterials with intrinsic osteoinductivity: geometric control of bone differentiation. Bone Engineering; Ed. J.M. Davies. Toronto: Em Squared Inc.

[17] Ruck J, Dahan-Oliel N, Montpetit K, Rauch F, Fassier F (2011) Fassier-Duval femoral rodding in children with osteogenesis imperfecta receiving bisphosphonates: functional outcomes at one year. *J. Child Orthop*. 5(3):217-224.

[18] Stockley I, Bell M, Sharrard WJ (1989) The role of expanding intramedullary rods in osteogenesis imperfecta. *J. Bone Joint Surg.* 71B:422–427.

[19] Sułko J, Radło W (2005) Operative management of long-bone of the upper limb in children with osteogenesis imperfecta. *Chir. Narzadow Ruchu Ortop. Pol.* 70:195–199.

[20] Zeitlin L, Fassier F, Glorieux FH (2003) Modern approach to children with osteogeneis imperfecta. *J. Pediatr Orthop.* 12B:77–87.

[21] Zionts LE, Ebramzadeh E, Stoot NS (1998) Complications in the use of the Bailey-Dubow extensible wire. *Clin. Orthop.* 18:102–109.

In: Combined Stimulating Methods …
Editor: Dmitry Popkov
ISBN: 978-1-63483-028-7

Chapter VI

USE OF INTRAMEDULLARY BIOACTIVE NAILING IN DEFORMITY CORRECTION IN PATIENTS WITH X-LINKED HEREDITARY HYPOPHOSPHATEMIC RICKETS

Arnold Popkov, PhD, MD*

Scientific and Clinical Laboratory for Deformity Correction and Limb Lengthening. Federal Russian State-Financed Ilizarov Scientific Center for Restorative Traumatology and Orthopaedics, Kurgan, Russia

ABSTRACT

Introduction. X-linked hereditary hypophosphatemic rickets (XHPR) is the most common form of the hypophosphatemic rickets caused by renal phosphate wasting. The operative procedures to correct multiplanar bone deformities may be indicated for prevention of secondary orthopedic complications.

The aim of this retrospective study was comparison of results of correction in short and long term follow-up in children with XHPR who underwent the treatment with either the Ilizarov device alone or a combined technique consisting of the Ilizarov fixator and FIN.

Material and methods. We retrospectively analyzed 47 cases of surgical treatment in children affected by XHPR. Simultaneous deformity

* Corresponding author: Ilizarov Scientific Center for Restorative Traumatology and Orthopaedics, 6, M.-Ulyanova Street, 640014 Kurgan, Russia; apopkov.46@mail.ru,

correction in femur and tibia was performed with the Ilizarov device (group I) or the combined method (group II).

Results. A monofocal bisegmental transosseous osteosynthesis was performed in group I on 24 limbs, a polyfocal bisegmental transosseous osteosynthesis was performed in 20 cases. In group II the monofocal polysegmental transosseous osteosynthesis was performed in 30 extremities, the polyfocal bisegmental – in 20 limbs.

The duration of external fixation was noted to be considerably shorter applying the combined technique: 124.7±14.9 days (group I) vs 87.4±13.2 days (group II).

In both groups deformity correction was achieved with a proper alignment and normal orientation of the knee joint. Nevertheless, while a child keep on growing in long term follow-up, deviations of the mechanic axis from the center of the knee joint have been developing again and values of mLDFA, mMPTA have become pathologic in the most of cases. In group I location of a newly developed deformity resembled to a preoperative one, i.e., both, diaphyseal and metaphyseal parts were deformed. It is worth of mentioning that in group II in all the cases an apex of deformity (CORA) was located in distal metadiaphyseal zone of the femur and proximal metadiaphyseal zone of the tibia. It is important that all of them in group II were out of zone of the intramedullary nail tracks, in other words it is possible to prevent deformity recurrence with FIN.

Conclusion. The deformities of lower limbs in children with XLHR should be operatively corrected. Application of a combined osteosynthesis allows to considerably reduce the duration of external fixation, decrease the number of infectious complications, avoid secondary displacement of fragments. There were no recurrent deformities in parts of bone reinforced by intramedullary nails.

Keywords: X-linked hereditary hypophosphatemic rickets, combined surgical technique

INTRODUCTION

X-linked hereditary hypophosphatemic rickets (XHPR) is the most common form of the hypophosphatemic rickets caused by renal phosphate wasting, impaired renal production of 1.25-dihydroxyvitamin D3 and abnormal bone mineralization [1,2,3]. Clinical orthopedic features become obvious since the beginning of ambulating and are manifested by varus or valgus deformities of the lower limb, torsion deformities, impaired gait, short stature, pathologic fractures [2,4,5,6]. The conservative treatment is not always successful. In such cases, operative procedures for correction multiplanar bone deformities may be indicated to prevent secondary orthopedic complications like pain, pathologic fractures, degenerative arthropathy; or for cosmetic reasons [7-9].

Patients with deformities have been treated by various methods of corrective osteotomy and fixation devices, such as Kirschner wires, plates, temporary epiphysiodesis, Ilizarov devices and intramedullary nailing devices [8,9-12]. Different problems related to surgical correction were reported, among them increased rate of non-union after osteotomies, delayed union, recurrent deformity, deep intramedullary infection, refracture, nerve palsy and pin tract infection [13-15].

In our opinion, the Ilizarov method remains the most efficient technique from the point of view of multi-planar and multi-apical deformity correction. Application of a circular external device is crucial for orthopedic surgeons in particular [8,11,12]. A combination of external fixation and intramedullary rigid osteosynthesis allows to reduce the period of external fixation [13]. Nevertheless, in pediatric practice such combination is not applicable; on the other hand, the deformity correction should be performed in childhood in order to prevent development of early arthrosis.

Results of deformity correction were compared in two groups of patients differentiated by use of the external fixator alone (group 1) and application of the combined technique (external fixator and intramedullary nails with bioactive coating, group 2). Criteria of comparison were efficiency of the procedure, duration of external fixation and occurred complications.

Material and Methods

We retrospectively analyzed 47 medical charts of children affected with XHPR and hospitalized for correction of developed deformities of the lower limb. Criteria of inclusion were: deformities of two segments (femur and tibia) on both limbs, age under 18 years old, simultaneous deformity correction in femur and tibia on one limb with the Ilizarov device (group I) or the combined method (the Ilizarov device and intramedullary nailing – group II).

Diagnostics of all the patients was based on the typical laboratory finding of hypophosphatemia, elevated alkaline phosphatase activity in combination with presence of limb deformities, low stature and beginning of deformity development in average at 2-year-old age.

All the children received adequate oral phosphate and calcitriol therapy. In all the cases drug-resistant deformities were detected, which induced the lower limb deformities requiring operative correction [9].

Criteria of assessment were as follows:

- mechanical axis deviation (MAD), mechanical lateral distal femoral angle (mLDFA), mechanical medial proximal tibial angle (mMPTA), angulations at a level of femoral and tibial diaphysis [15,16], torsions;
- type of operation, number and levels of osteotomies, immediate or gradual character of corrections;
- duration of the external osteosynthesis;
- complications, their outcome;
- classification of results according to Lascombes [17] was used in 10-12 months after treatment.

Weight bearing full-length anteroposterior radiographs of the entire lower extremities were taken in a standing position with the patella centered forward, and lateral radiographs of each segment with adjacent joints were obtained. Radiologic indices (MAD, mMPTA, mLDFA) were measured preoperatively, after frame removal and in 10-12 months after treatment.

Surgical correction procedures were planned according to the patient's clinical assessment and radiographic data. Principles of deformity correction with the Ilizarov fixator considering CORA and ACA were strictly respected in all cases [12,16]. Taking into consideration systemic involvement of limbs, i.e. there were no intact limb for reference in planning of the correction gain, the average statistic radiologic values normal for the age were used [15].

The first surgical step was standard in both groups: it consisted of application of the external fixator, followed by percutaneous osteotomies. Frame assembly (rings and half-rings), position of olive wires and hinge elements were dictated by anatomic location and severity of the deformities in both groups. If the deformity was located at only one level of the bone segment, one single osteotomy was performed through a 10–15 mm longitudinal incision centered over the metaphyseal, metadiaphyseal or diaphyseal region. If the deformities were more severe, the double percutaneous osteotomies were done. In tibia the osteotomy of the fibula was performed in the lower third or between the middle-lower thirds of the shaft.

In all the cases the operation was performed on both segments of the lower limb simultaneously under one general anesthesia.

In group II the second step was FIN with chitosan-hydroxyapatite (HA)-coated titanium nails. In cases of monofocal correction two entry holes at metaphysis level were created with an awl in an oblique direction toward the osteotomy, at some distance from the growth plate. We recommend to select the closest metaphysis to the osteotomy in order to facilitate insertion of the intramedullary nails and proper orientation after intraoperative correction. The 1.8–2 mm nails were contoured to achieve a curvature of about 50–60°. Nails must be carefully advanced one at a time following the natural bow of the diaphysis, pushed across the osteotomy site and directed to the opposite metaphysis. After the nails have been inserted, they were reoriented so, that their concavities were oriented toward the convexity of the deformity. Once the nails were in place, the deformities were immediately corrected - totally or partially depending on the angulation. Generally, the acute total correction was used in deformities inferior to 30°. Obviously, a proper FIN construct facilitated realignment and prevented undesirable displacement of bone fragments. The free ends of nails were bent outside the bone to prevent migration during realignment. Then, they were trimmed, leaving approximately 5–10 mm from the bone surface. The skin was closed in one layer.

In cases of bifocal correction of a complex deformity, bipolar combined FIN was more appropriate. The intramedullary nails were inserted towards each other from opposite metaphyses. This principal of FIN positioning was used in diseases associated with extreme bone fragility or in bifocal limb lengthening [18,19]. Insertion and orientation of intramedullary nails were performed according to the above mentioned steps.

Finally, the additional wires/half-pins were inserted with the FIN construct in place: in the proximal and distal rings (short arches) and/or some middle-ring wires in bifocal correction.

Corrections of angular and rotational deformities were performed either in the acute or the gradual setting, depending on the severity of the deformity. Deformities of 30° and more were corrected partially at once, residual deformities – gradually. In case of gradual correction the lengthening of 1-2 cm was gained. Gradual correction can be initiated on the 5th postoperative day. In all cases we strived to eliminate the present deformities and to prevent under- or overcorrection, which is known to be fraud with relapse of deformations [7,10]. Once the external fixator has been removed, regenerates remained protected by at least one intramedullary nail in group II. In all the patients of group II the intramedullary nails stayed in their place for the whole follow-up period. By the end of operative treatment all the patients continued receiving oral phosphate and calcitriol therapy.

RESULTS

The mean age of patients in group I was 10.7±2.4 years, in the group II - 8.9±2.1 years. In both groups varus limb deformity was more frequent: 40 limbs in the first group and 46 – in the second. Valgus deformity was faced only in 4 patients, 2 in each group.

Considering the location of deformities, the monofocal bisegmental transosseous osteosynthesis (one osteotomy of femur and one of tibia) was performed in group 1 on 24 limbs, a polyfocal (double osteotomy of at least one of the segments) bisegmental transosseous osteosynthesis was performed in 20 cases. In group 2 the monofocal polysegmental transosseous osteosynthesis was performed on 30 extremities, polyfocal bisegmental – in 20 limbs (figures 38 and 39).

Duration of the external fixation period with the traditional Ilizarov technique vs HA-coated titanium nails is presented in table 6.1. It is obvious that the duration of external fixation in group 2 was considerably shorter, which can be explained by stimulation of bone formation by means of bioactive implans in the osteotomy site [26-28].

Table 6.1. Duration of the external fixation (days)

	Group I	Group II
Varus deformity of lower limb	124.7±14.9	87.4±13.2*
Valgus deformity of lower limb	137.8±13.6	111.3±7.4*

*Significant difference (P<0.05, Student t test) in comparison with the group I.

Table 6.2 presents values of MAD, mLDFA, mMPTA before treatment, after frame removal, by the beginning of weight-bearing and in a year follow-up.

Table 6.2. Values of MAD, mLDFA, mMPTA

		Before traitement			At the beginning of full weight bearing after frame removal			In 10-12 months after frame removal		
		MAD	mLDFA	mMPTA	MAD	mLDFA	mMPTA	MAD	mLDFA	mMPTA
Group 1	Initial varus deformity of limb	40.8±9.95	100.5±3.8	77.7±3.5	0.9±4.0	88.2±1.6	89.3±1.7	11.5±5.3	92.5±11.3	88.1±7.3
	Initial valgus deformity of limb	39.8±4.1	68.5±2.6	103.3±3.5	5.1±0.96	89±1.8	92±1.6	6.7±3.1	8.9±7.5	91.3±5.3
Group 2	Initial varus deformity of limb	40.2±9.2	100.4±3.9	77.1±3.8	0.7±3.9	88.6±1.6	89.3±2.1	4.9±8.2	90.1±6.1	89.1±7.9
	Initial valgus deformity of limb	42.5±4.9	67.3±1.7	106.3±3.1	3.3±1.3	88.3±0.5	89.8±0.96	5.6±2.9	87.3±7.5	89.6±10.2

In both groups deformity correction was achieved with a proper alignment and normal orientation of the knee space according to mechanic axes of segments. The results of correction remained preserved during the first year after treatment.

The following complications were observed in group I: pin track infection in 24 cases (in 4 cases it required changing of wires under general anesthesia); transient sciatic or peroneal nerve palsy - 6 cases; displacement of bone fragments in postoperative period requiring adjustment of the Ilizarov fixator under general anesthesia – 8 cases; in 2 cases a plastic deformity at a level of correction occurred during the first week after frame removal, it required redressment of the deformity under general anesthesia and immobilization in a new plaster cast. In group II pin track infection was noted in 16 cases (in two cases wires were removed and reinserted); 7 cases of sciatic or peroneal nerve palsy with complete regression; in two cases intramedullary nails were insufficiently cut off and their free ends irritated soft tissues. Thus, the results in group I were classified according to Lascombes [18] as follows: category I in deformity correction – 30 extremities, IIa – 12 limbs, IIb – 2 limbs. In group II : I – 46 limbs, IIa – 4 limbs. It is worth of mentioning that complications with sequelae (III, IV categories) were not observed in any patient of both groups.

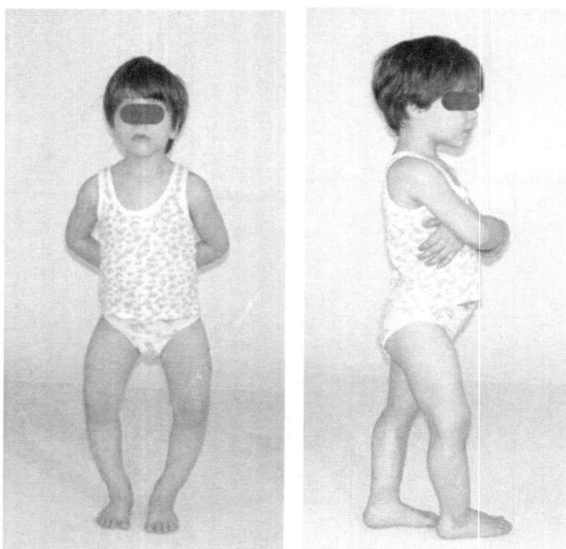

(a) (b)

Figure 38. (Continued).

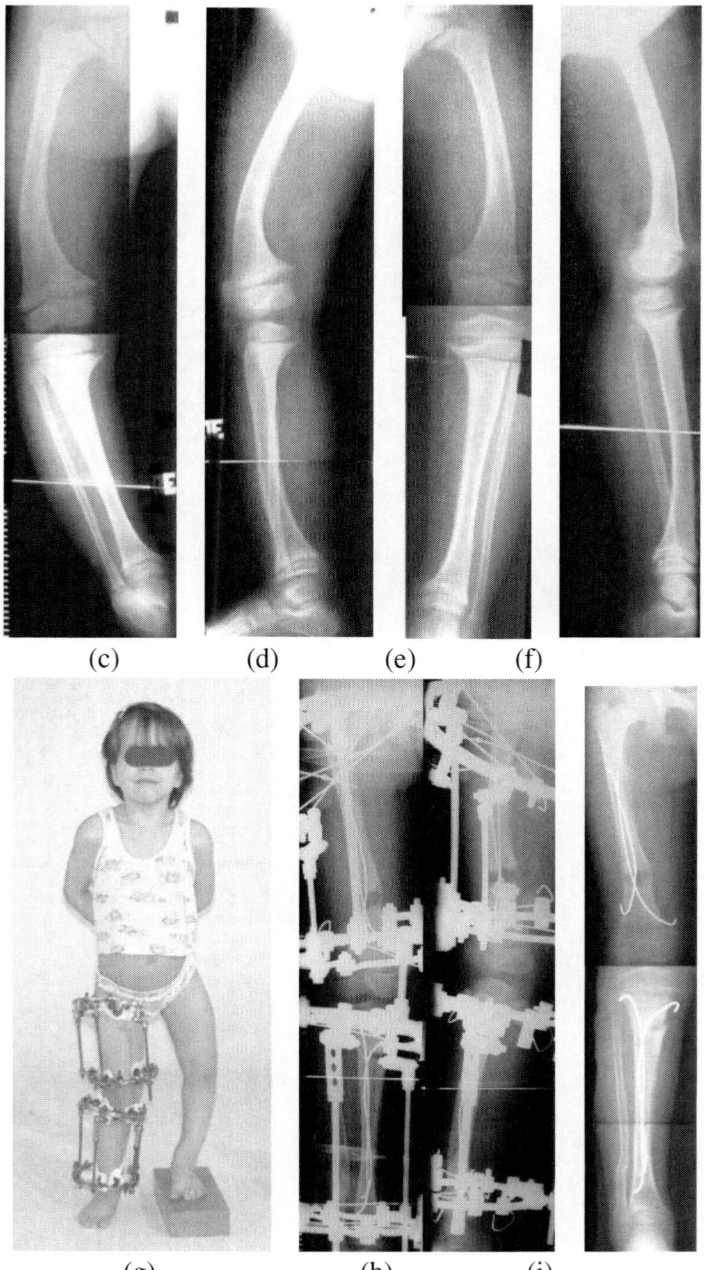

Figure 38. (Continued).

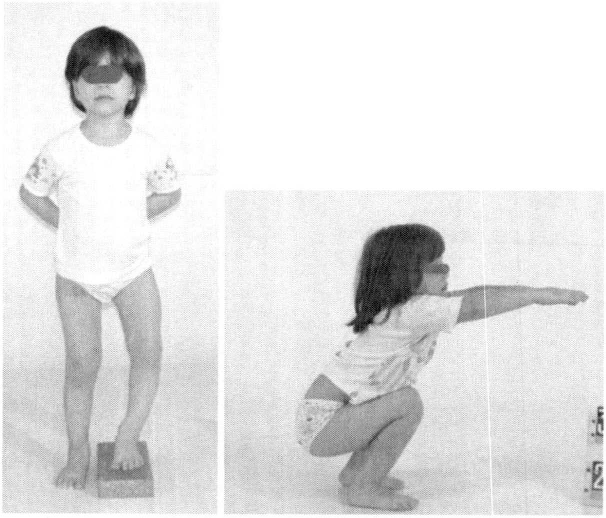

(j) (k)

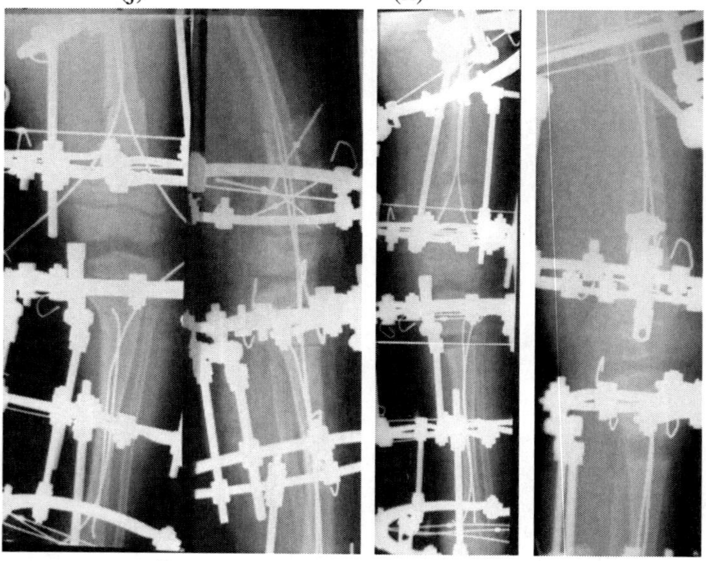

(l) (m) (n)

Figure 38. (Continued).

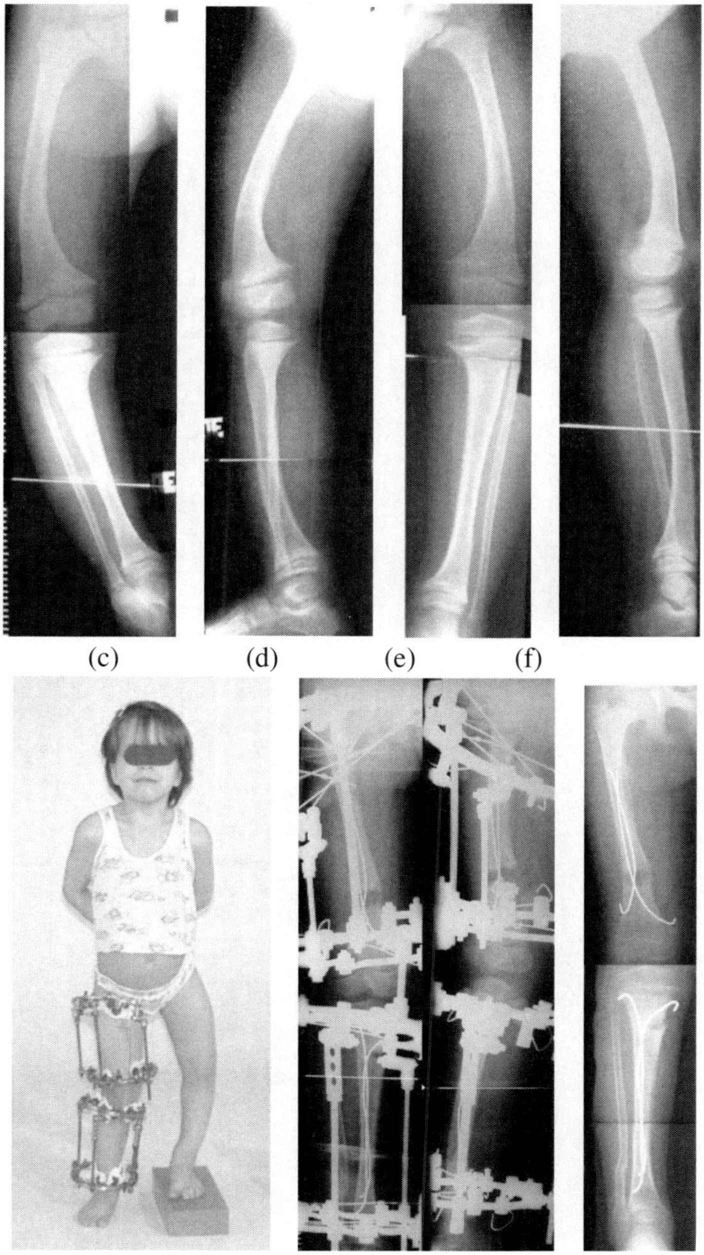

(c) (d) (e) (f)

(g) (h) (i)

Figure 38. (Continued).

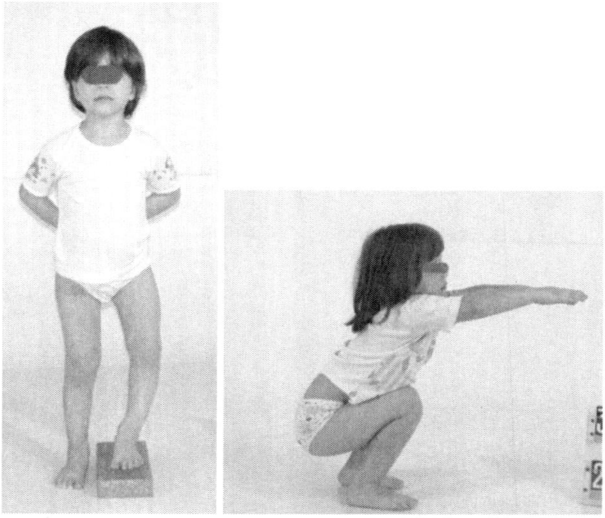

(j) (k)

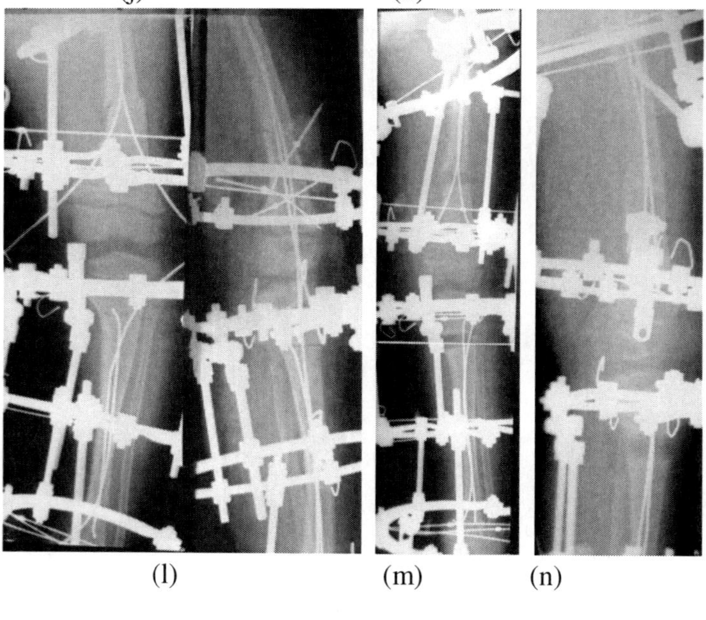

(l) (m) (n)

Figure 38. (Continued).

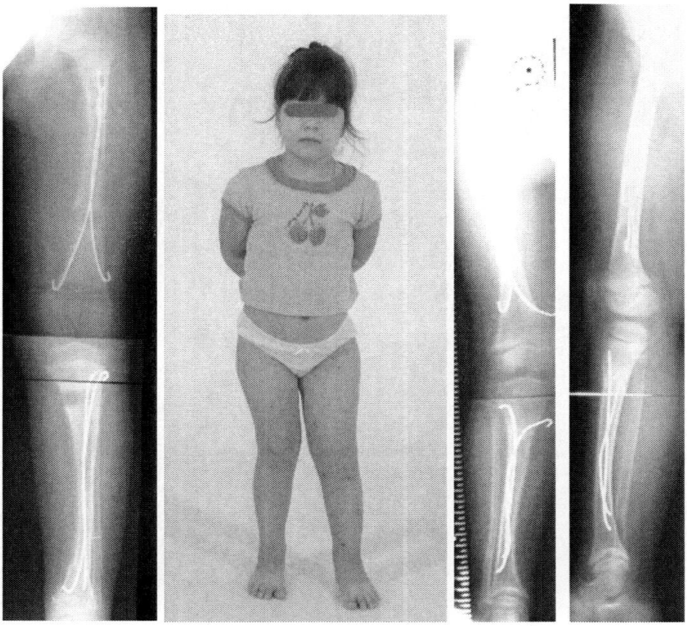

(o) (p) (q) (r)

Figure 38. A 5-year-old girl with hypophosphatemic rickets. Before surgery: clinical appearance (a,b); AP and lateral X-rays, right side (c,d), left side (e,f). Ilizarov fixator in place for multisegmental correction of the right lower limb : clinical appearance (g), X-rays (h). Note the orientation of intramedullary nails to counter varus forces. View of the right lower limb 2 weeks after removal of the external fixator: biomechanical axis of the lower extremity was restored (i). Clinical appearance 1 year after removal of the external fixator (right side) and before surgery of the left lower limb (j,k). Surgical treatment of the left lower limb ; intraoperative X-ray immediately after insertion of intramedullary nails (l), AP and lateral X-rays: combined multisegmental external fixation/flexible intramedullary nailing (FIN). The biomechanical axis of the lower extremity was restored (m,n). X-ray of the left lower limb 10 days after removal of the external fixator (o). Patient 1 year after removal of the external fixator (left side) (p). Fixation period for the left side was 48 days. X-rays of the right lower limb 1 year after removal of the external fixator. Axial alignment still satisfactory (q,r). *NB! This figure has been originally published in Flexible Intramedullary Nailing in Children. 2010, pp 291-299 Use of FIN for Correction of Deformities in Children with Familial Hypophosphatemic Rickets Author: Dimitri Popkov © Springer-Verlag Berlin Heidelberg 2010 Material Requested: Fig.23.1 p. 292 With kind permission of Springer Science+Business Media.*

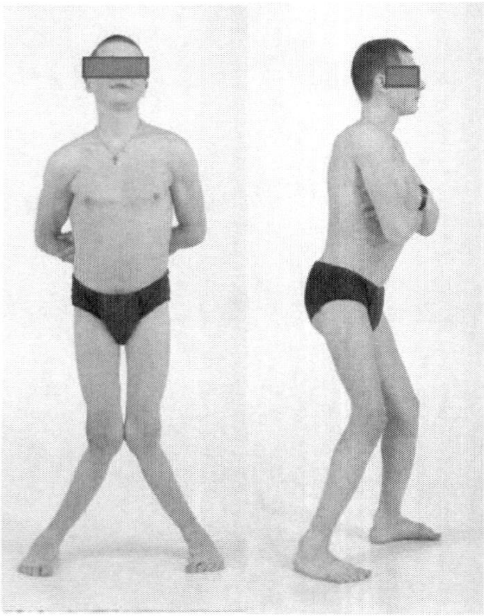

(a)

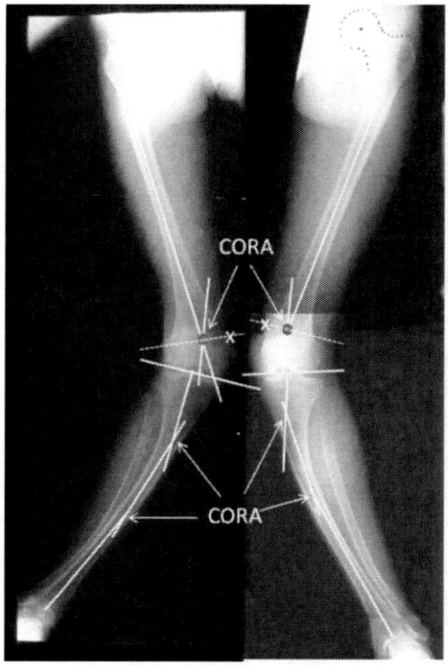

(b)

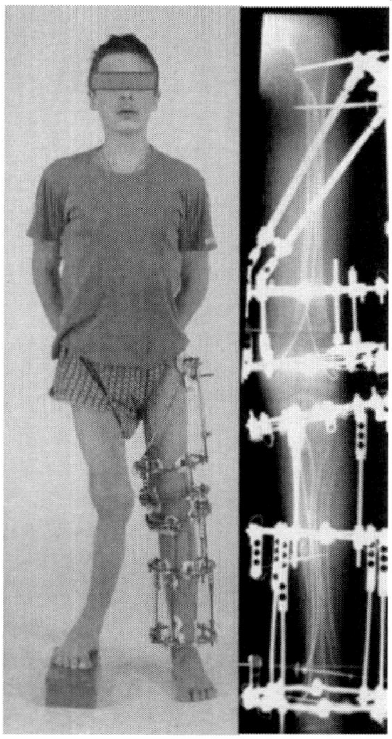

(c)

Figure 39. (Continued).

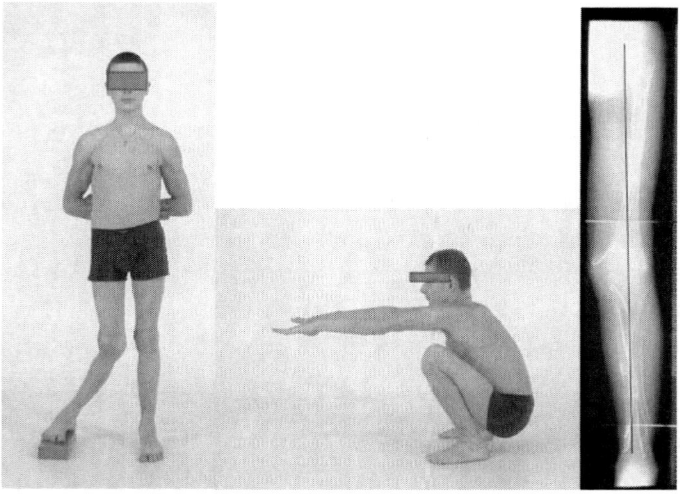

(d)

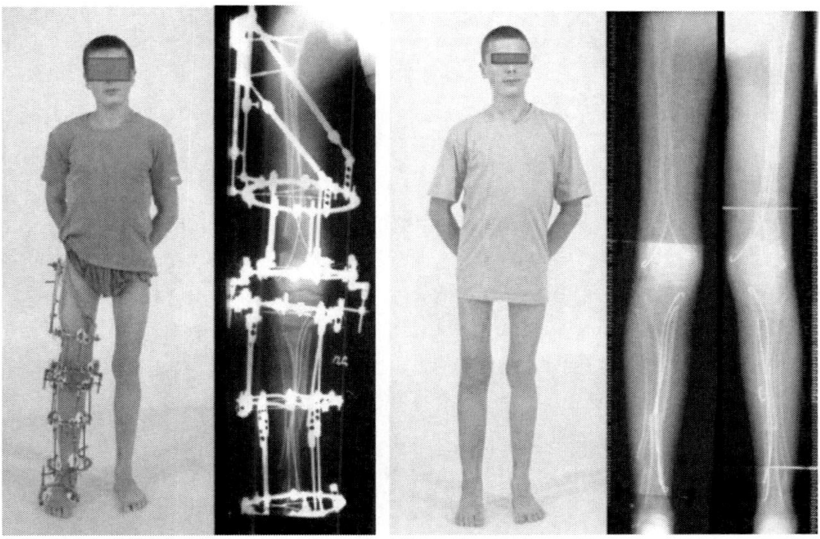

(e) (f)

Figure 39. A 17-year-old boy with hypophosphatemic rickets. Before surgery: clinical appearance (a); AP X-rays, illustration of preoperative planning, defining CORA and ACA (axis of correction of angulation, marked X) (b); Ilizarov fixator in place for multisegmental correction of the left lower limb : clinical appearance and, X-rays, duration of external fixation 91 days (c); clinical appearance et X-rays 1 year after removal of the external fixator (left side) and before surgery of the right lower limb (d); Ilizarov fixator in place for multisegmental correction of the right lower limb : clinical appearance and, X-rays, duration of external fixation 97 days (e); clinical appearance and X-rays 1 month after frame removal (f).

DISCUSSION

Orthopedic complications of the X-linked hereditary hypophosphatemic rickets - severe deformities of lower limbs – develop in young age, so indications for operative treatment appear rather early [2,5,20]. Series of studies were published describing performed surgical treatment even when a patient's resistance to conservative treatment was stated [5,8,10]. Studies revealed that excess of fibroblast growth factor 23 action results in hypophosphatemic disease because it suppresses the expression of sodium-phosphate cotransporters in the proximal tubules of kidneys, which mediate physiological phosphate reabsorption [21-23]. Imel et al. [3] discovered a significant increasing of circulating FGF23 concentrations while phosphate and calcitriol therapy, which can be a cause of resistance of patients with X-linked hereditary hypophosphatemic rickets to conservative treatment.

The developed deformities of lower limbs should be surgically corrected in order to maintain normal biomechanic conditions for ambulating, for cosmetic reasons and to prevent early severe arthrosis of hip and knee joints [12,13,23].

Various methods are used for fixation of bone fragments after performed osteotomies as plaster cast, K-wires, bone plates, external fixators, intramedullary nails [4,5,7,9,10,12]. It goes without saying that application of intramedullary locked nails in pediatric orthopedics is restricted.

Circular devices of external fixation with parallel or hexapodal position of connecting rods [8,11,13] provide the best conditions from the point of view of accuracy of deformity correction, abilities of gradual controlled correction of all deformity components in a postoperative period at a level of femur and tibia simultaneously, absence of interference in growth cartilages, absence of inhibition of the following segment growth in length.

In our study in both groups of patients the required correction was achieved simultaneously in femur and in tibia using the Ilizarov fixator and principles of Ilizarov method. Difference between the groups was in duration of fixation, number and severity of complications.

A general problem of external fixation remains a long period of fixation: from 4 months or 146 days in average [8,11] to 6 months [7]. There is a possibility to reduce considerably the duration of external fixation reported by Kocaoglu et al. [5]. The external device was removed either after acute correction and introducing the intramedullary nail or by the end of distraction period. That approach allowed to reduce the duration of external fixation considerably, to prevent recurrent deformities and to preserve the accuracy of correction peculiar to application of circular fixators [12,13,15]. But the application of locked intramedullary nails is inadvisable in children and it requires another approach.

Considering advantages of FIN [18,19,24], we applied this type of osteosynthesis with elastic intramedullary nails coated with a bioactive layer in children affected by XHPR, who underwent acute correction on femur and tibia. It allowed to decrease the mean duration of external fixation to 87.4 days in deformity correction in varus limb axis and to 111.3 days in valgus limb axis (in average by 37 and 26 days correspondingly).

A prolonged period of external fixation can be associated with a high risk of complications. Petje et al. [8] reported about one episode minimum of infectious complication around wires or half-pins in every patient while deformity correction with an external fixator. Song et al. [13] noted in 20 patients 18 major complications (recurrent deformity, fracture after frame removal, peroneal nerve palsy) and 13 minor complications. In the series of Fucentese et al. [7] development of contractures of the knee joint and infection were observed.

In our study the FIN application allowed to decrease infectious complications and to avoid any secondary displacement of bone fragments during gradual correction, fractures and deformities at the level of correcting osteotomies after removal of external fixators. No complications concerning migration of intramedullary nails with bioactive coating were also noted.

In general, a high rate of deformity relapse is observed during the long term follow-up after operative correction in children with this pathology. Song et al. [13] observed complications (recurrent deformity or fracture at a level of correction) in 10 patients out of 21, Rubinovitch et al. [4] reported relapse of deformity in 27% of cases. Petje et al. [8] observed up to 90% of recurrent deformities after primary correction and up to 60% after secondary surgeries, besides the rate of relapses reduced after the age of 14 years old. There is no data yet of development or relapse of the deformity of lower limbs in long term follow up (5-7 years) after surgical correction of deformities in children with XHPR and after the end of natural growth. It requires a longer period of follow up.

CONCLUSION

Nevertheless, advantages of combined osteosynthesis (circular external fixator and FIN with bioactive coating) can be already stated as shorter duration of external fixation, decrease of infectious complications and absence of secondary displacement of fragments during correction or deformities at the osteotomy level after frame removal.

REFERENCES

[1] Albright F, Butler AM, Bloomberg E (1937) Rickets resistant to vitamin D therapy. *Am. J. Dis. Child.* 54:529-547.

[2] Cho HY, Lee BH, Knag JH, Ha IS, Cheong HI, Choi Y (2005) A clinical and molecular genetic study of hypophosphatemic rickets in children. *Pediatr Res.* 58:329–333.

[3] Imel EA, DiMeglio LA, Hui SL, Carpenter TO, Econs MJ (2010) Treatement of X-linked hypophosphatemia with calcitriol and phosphate increases circulating fibroblast growth factor 23 concentrations. *J. Clin. Endocrinol. Metab.* 95(4):1846-1859.

[4] Rubinovitch M, Said SE, Glorieux FH, Cruess RL, Rogala E (1988) Principles and results of corrective lower limb osteotomies for patients with vitamin D-resistant hypophosphatemic rickets. *Clin. Orthop Relat.* Res. 237:264–270.

[5] Kocaoglu M, Bilen FE, Sen C, Eralp L, Balci HI (2011) Combined technique for the correction of lower-limb deformities resulting from metabolic bone disease. *J. Bone Joint Surg. Br.* 93(1):52-56.

[6] Zivičnjak M, Schnabel D, Billing H, Staude H, Filler G, Querfeld U, Schumacher M, Pyper A, Schröder C, Brämswig J, Haffner D (2011) Hypophosphatemic Rickets Study Group of the "Arbeitsgemeinschaft für Pädiatrische Endokrinologie" and "Gesellschaft für Pädiatrische Nephrologie". Pediatr Nephrol. Age-related stature and linear body segments in children with X-linked hypophosphatemic rickets. 26(2):223-231.

[7] Fucentese SF, Neuhaus TJ, Ramseier LE, Ulrich Exner G (2008) Metabolic and orthopedic management of X-linked vitamin D-resistant hypophosphatemic rickets. *J. Child Orthop.* 2:285-291.

[8] Petje G, Meizer R, Radler C, Aigner N, Grill F (2008) Deformity correction in children with hereditary hypophosphatemic rickets. *Clin. Orthop. Relat. Res.* 466:3078-3085.

[9] Evans GA, Arulanantham K, Gage JR (1980) Primary hypophosphatemic rickets: effect of oral phosphate and vitamin D on growth and surgical treatment. *J. Bone Joint Surg. Am.* 62:1130–1138.

[10] Eyres KS, Brown J, Douglas DL (1993) Osteotomy and intramedullary nailing for the correction of progressive deformity in vitamin D-resistant hypophosphataemic rickets. *J. R. Coll. Surg. Edinb*.38:50–54.

[11] Matsubara H, Tsuchiya H, Kabata T, Sakurakichi K, Watanabe K, Tomita K (2008) Deformity correction for vitamin D-resistant hypophosphatemic rickets of adults. *Arch. Orthop. Trauma Surg*. 128(10):1137-1143.

[12] Choi IH, Kim JK, Chung CY, Cho TJ, Lee SH, Suh SW, Whang KS, Park HW, Song KS (2002) Deformity correction of knee and leg lengthening by Ilizarov method in hypophosphatemic rickets: outcomes and significance of serum phosphate level. *J. Pediatr Orthop*. 22(5):626-631.

[13] Song HR, Soma Raju VV, Kumar S, Lee SH, Suh SW, Kim JR, Hong JS. Deformity correction by external fixation and/or intramedullary nailing in hypophosphatemic rickets (2006) *Acta Orthop*. 77(2):307-314.

[14] Ferris B, Walker C, Jackson A, Kirwan E (1991) The orthopaedic management of hypophosphataemic rickets. *J. Pediatr Orthop*. 11(3):367–373.

[15] Popkov D, Lascombes P, Berte N, Hetzel L, Ribeiro Baptista B, Popkov A, Journeau P (2015) The normal radiological anteroposterior alignment of lower limb in children. *Skeletal Radiol*. 44(2):197-206.

[16] Paley D, Herzenberg JE, Tetsworth K, McKie J, Bhave A (1994) Deformity planing for frontal and sagittal plan corrective osteotomies. *Orthop. Clin. North Am*. 25:425–465.

[17] Lascombes P, Popkov D, Huber H, Haumont T, Journeau P (2012) Classification of complications after progressive long bone lengthening: proposal for a new classification. *Orthop. Traumatol. Surg. Res*. 98(6):629-637.

[18] Popkov D, Popkov A, Haumont T, Journeau P, Lascombes P (2010). Flexible intramedullary nail use in limb lengthening. *J. Pediatr Orthop*. 30:910-18.

[19] Lascombes P. Flexible Intramedullary Nailing in Children: *The Nancy University Manual* (2010) Springer.

[20] Petersen DJ, Boniface AM, Schranck FW, Rupich RC, Whyte MP (1992) X-linked hypophosphatemic rickets: a study (with literature review) of linear growth response to calcitriol and phosphate therapy. *J. Bone Miner Res*. 7(6):583–597.

[21] Ozono K. Bone and joint diseases in children (2010) Phosphaturic hormone, FGF23 and bone metabolism. *Clin Calcium*. 20(6):896-903.

[22] Shimada T, Yamazaki Y,Takahashi M, Hasegawa H et al. (2005) Vitamin D receptor-independent FGF23 actions in regulating phosphate and vitamin D metabolism. *Am. J. Physiol. Renal Physol.* 289(5):1088-1095.

[23] Larson AN, Trousdale RT, Pagnano MW, Hanssen AD, Lewallen DG, Sanchez-Sotelo J (2010) Hip and knee arthroplasty in hypophosphatemic rickets. *J. Arthroplasty.* 25(7):1099-1103.

[24] Popkov D, Journeau P, Popkov A, Haumont T, Lascombes P (2010) Ollier's disease limb lenghtening: Should intramedullary nailing be combined with circular external fixation? *Orthop. Traumatol. Surg. Res.* 96:348—353.

[25] Chatelet JC, Setiey L (2004) Comportement osseux à long terme après implantation d'un pivot fémoral totalement revêtu d'hydroxyapatite. *Rev Chir. Orthop Reparatrice Appar Mot.* 90(7):628-635.

[26] Popkov D (2010) Use of FIN for correction of deformities in children with familial hypophosphatemic rickets. In : Lascombes P. Flexible Intramedullary Nailing in Children. Springer. pp291-299.

[27] Harrell RM, Lyles KW, Harrelson JM, Friedman NE, Drezner MK (1985) Healing of bone disease in X-linked hypophosphatemic rickets/osteomalacia: induction and maintenance with phosphorus and calcitriol. *J. Clin. Invest.* 75:1858–1868.

In: Combined Stimulating Methods …
Editor: Dmitry Popkov
ISBN: 978-1-63483-028-7

Chapter VII

Hybrid Technologies in Spinal Deformity Surgery

Sergey Ryabykh**, *PhD, MD
Clinical Laboratory of Axial skeleton,
Federal Russian State-Financed Ilizarov Scientific Center for Restorative Traumatology and Orthopaedics, Kurgan, Russia

Abstract

Chapter V is a review of contemporary techniques of osteosynthesis of the spine. Advantages and disadvantages of modern internal systems of spinal correction and fixation are assessed, variants of combination of external and internal osteosynthesis of the spine are presented. There will be demonstrated variants, methodology and advantages of state-to-art methods of external spinal fixation and combined approaches associating merits of the external fixation and Cotrel-Dubousset systems. Abilities and advantages of the technique are analyzed and clinical observations with analysis of efficiency of correction are presented.

Keywords: Combined technique, spine surgery

* Corresponding author: Ilizarov Scientific Center for Restorative Traumatology and Orthopaedics, 6, M.-Ulyanova Street, 640014 Kurgan, Russia; rso_@mail.ru.

Introduction

Spinal deformity is one of the most frequent and leading syndrome of complex vertebrogenic pathology, congenital anomalies of vertebrae and ribs, systemic and neuromuscular diseases, posttraumatic modifications, idiopathic scoliosis and often their combination. The most important features of spinal deformity are the rate of progression and amount of deformity. These same features influence on cosmetic and functional outcome and, as a result, on quality and length of life.

Surgical treatment of patients with a spinal deformity is supposed to solve the following problems: to stop deformity progression, to perform its maximum possible correction and to provide conditions for preserving the result. Despite of various manifestations of the disease, patients with spinal deformities are united by one common group of problems, they are variability of neurologic deficit, body balance disorder, persistent progression, functional degradation of cardiopulmonary system, unsatisfactory appearance and low quality of patients' life [2, 7, 8, 9]. Surgical treatment of patients with deformities over 100° is characterized by a high intraoperative risk and a high rate of complications in the postoperative period [2, 9, 10, 11].

All the methods used for spinal deformity correction can be subdivided in 2 groups: basic techniques, i.e., standard techniques of acute correction using widely spread implants; hybrid approach, i.e., combination of mobilizing methods (variants of traction and methods of vertebrotomy) with methods of distraction, derotation and reclination (in kyphosis) by means of external and internal fixation devices.

This chapter deals with indications and techniques of external fixation in children and adults, their combination with methods of spine mobilization in severe deformities and internal instrumental fixation. In severe forms of idiopathic scoliosis in children it is conventional to use tactics of preliminary traction for spine deformity correction, cranio- or halo-pelvic traction or traction with external fixation systems. Application of methods of preoperative halo-traction allows manipulating the major deformity arch indirectly by means of the most mobile spine regions, that considerably reduces this influence [3, 11]. Systems of external transpedicular fixation remain applicable, they possess mechanical advantage from the point of view of application of corrective efforts to major deformity arch while gradual correction, preserving patient's mobility and monitoring of neurologic and somatic status of the patient [1, 4, 5, 6, 10].

Despite many unsolved problems for the moment, we have tried to disclose the author's view on tactical issues of surgical treatment, such as possibility to perform simultaneously a neurosurgical and vertebrologic stages, a type of fixation, its extension, indications and techniques of combining of instrumentation methods, indications and application possibilities for corrective and shortening vertebrotomies. Also, the treatment outcome and complications are analyzed.

METHODS OF EXTERNAL FIXATION

Halo-pelvic System

One of the most expanded types of spinal external fixation is halo-pelvic traction. The method is widely used for correction of severe spinal deformities of any etiology, including atypical (cervical and cervical-thoracic) locations. In our practice, we use this technique independently. The technique is applied as a variant of traction during the first stage of surgical correction, it is also combined with methods of mobilization of the major arch. The second stage is transpedicular fixation of the spine. Besides, this technique is used as a variant of a "lifeboat" in pressure sores at the apex of kyphosis of any etiology. The variant of extrafocal fixation allows to create a reserve of soft tissues for wound healing by means of stabilization and distraction efforts [3].

The device is applied to the patient lying in the supine position under general anesthesia with. Primary distraction for construction tension is performed on the operating table. Then starting from the 2nd day of the postoperative period the distraction along the axial rods is administrated at the rate of 0.5 cm per day within 7-21 days. Dressing with monitoring of wounds is performed in two days. The time of traction is determined empirically according to rigidity of the deformity and degree of the device tension. The traction longer than 3 weeks is not recommended because of the risk of infection complications. During the distraction period the patients can take care of themselves independently, clinical control of neurologic and somatic complications is extremely important. If the latter ones occurred, the distraction efforts are reduced by 1-2 cm following by dorsal transpedicular fixation.

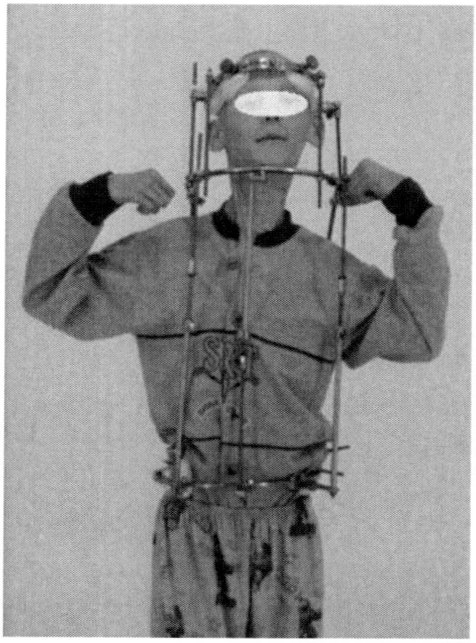

Figure 40. Patient's image after deformity correction by Ilizarov halo-pelvic system.

The halo-pelvic device is assembled of Ilizarov set components (Figure 40) or the module halo-pelvic apparatus is applied (Patent RF utility model N 124137 dtd 20.01.2013) (Figure 41).

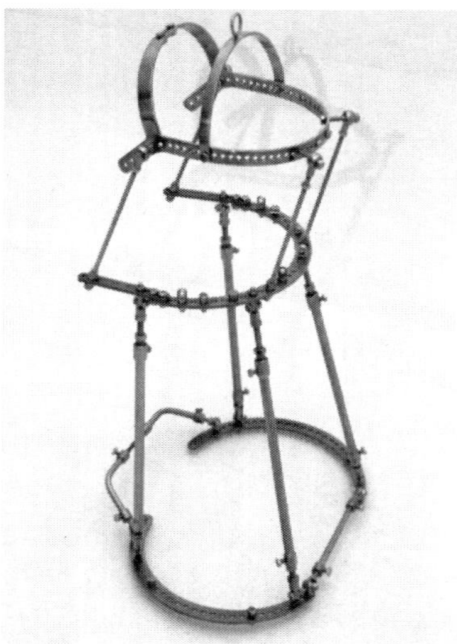

Figure 41. Halo-pelvic apparatus of the module type.

Device for the External Transpedicular Fixation

This type of external fixation is used in spinal deformities over 100° of thoracic and lumbar location, as well as in inflammatory processes of soft tissues of the back on the background of unstable lesions of vertebrae [5, 6]. It is not used independently, it is applied as a traction technique to prepare to dorsal instrumental fixation.

The surgery is performed under narcosis with the patient in the prone position. The frame assembling depends on the amount and 3D orientation of deformity arches. Threaded rods are inserted by pairs into the vertebra arch pedicles through the micro incisions up to 0.5 cm. They form support units (Figure 42a). Every unit contains 3-4 segments depending on anatomical features of the patient's spine. If fixation of the pelvis is required, two pairs of threaded rods are inserted in the wings of iliac bones bilaterally.

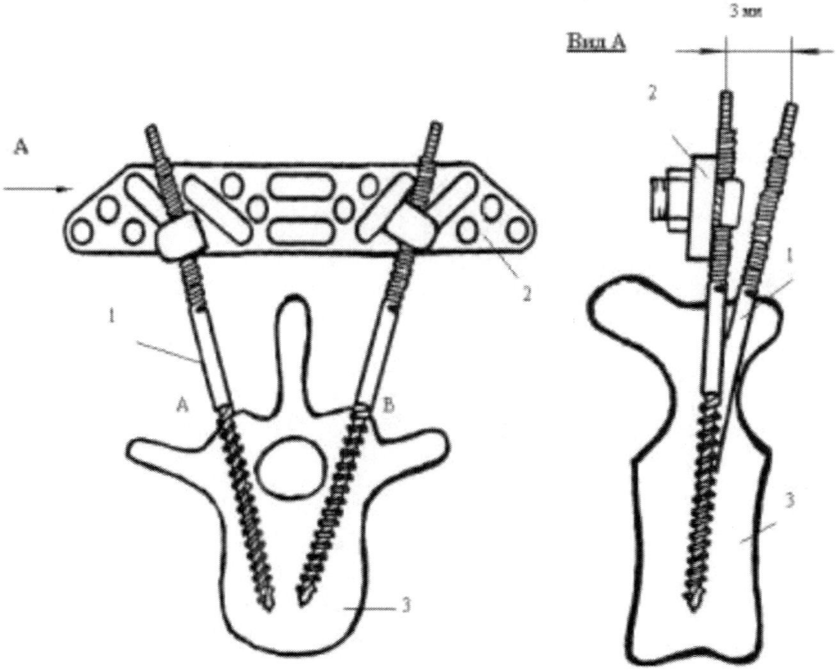

Figure 42. Assembling stages of the device for external fixation in severe idiopathic scoliosis (Lenke 3C+): insertion scheme of Schanz screws (a), connection of support units (b).

Then units are connected with longitudinal rods. Partial acute correction of the spinal deformity is performed on the operating table followed by antiseptic dressing (Figure 42b). Maximum possible correction of the spine is achieved during the postoperative period with monitoring of the neurologic status and X-ray control.

Dressings are changed every 3rd day. By the end of 10-14 days of correction in the frame at the rate of 0.5 cm/day the final open transpedicular instrumental correction and fixation of achieved spinal deformity correction is performed simultaneously with formation of posterior spondilodesis. This technique provides good and satisfactory treatment results (correction over 70%) minimizing the risk of neurologic and somatic complications.

External Transpedicular – Pelvic Fixation

Combined technique is also used as a lifeboat technology in inflammatory processes of soft tissues at the deformity apex of the lumbar spine. The technique unites advantages of transpedicular spinal fixation with pelvic screw fixation and localizes mechanical efforts in the lumber department. Besides, the technique can be used as preparation for the major stage of correction.

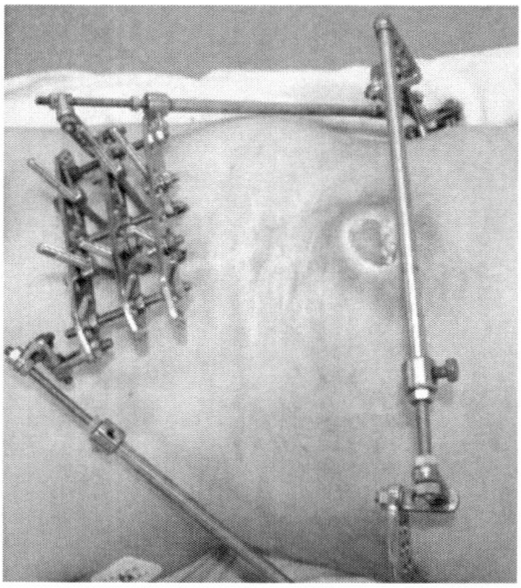

Figure 43. External transpedicular-pelvic fixation as a method of extrafocal fixation for pressuresore healing at the apex of deformity in congenital kyphosis on the myelocele background in a 9-year-old female.

The surgery is performed from a dorsal approach. Administration of narcosis and assembling of units don't vary. A distinctive feature is assembling of a transversal rod between pelvic units and their connection by two longitudinal rods with a spinal unit. It allows to build a united trapeze of rigidity (Figure 43). Dressing mode and distraction rate are the same.

COMBINED METHODS

Combination of Halo-pelvic and Posterior Instrumental Fixation

"Connector"- type systems are used in actively growing children. This method is favorable for patients with severe spinal deformity and high risk of somatic and neurologic complications [11]. The external fixation is aimed to control somatic and neurologic status.

Let us review this technique on the example of a patient with severe progressing cervical-thoracic scoliosis in systemic pathology, who has not received an adequate well-timed orthopedic care for a long period. By the age of 11 he was already affected by serious stato-dynamic and functional disorders, which impair his life quality and even threaten his life. Obviously, the very patient's existence was challenged without solving the orthopedic problem.

The male patient, 11 years old, was first seen for spinal deformity by a spinal surgeon in July 2011. The anamnesis revealed that the patient has been followed by an orthopedists since the age of one, when the deformities of limbs appeared. He was administrated a conventional treatment as massage of limbs and orthopedic shoes. The diagnosis of Ollier disease was verified by geneticist in 2001. The spinal deformity has been persisting for the last 2 years. Orthopaedic status showed disproportionate stature, evident cachexia with a weight of 18 kg, decompensated rigid extended right-side cervico-thoracic scoliosis with deviated torso to the right and head to the left up to 90° of Cobb's angle, gibbus on the right, hypertrophic muscles of the neck being more severe on the right, clinodactyly and hypertrophied phalanges of the fingers, and grade I funnel chest deformity (Figure 44 a,b). The traction test proved apparent rigidity of the deformity. Minimal exercise (walk up to 20 m distance) caused growing respiratory insufficiency. The lower limbs muscle strength in neurologic status was reduced to 3 according to ASIA score. No sensory impairment and pelvic organ dysfunction were detected. The patient developed quick fatigue with episodes of hypoxia (falling asleep).

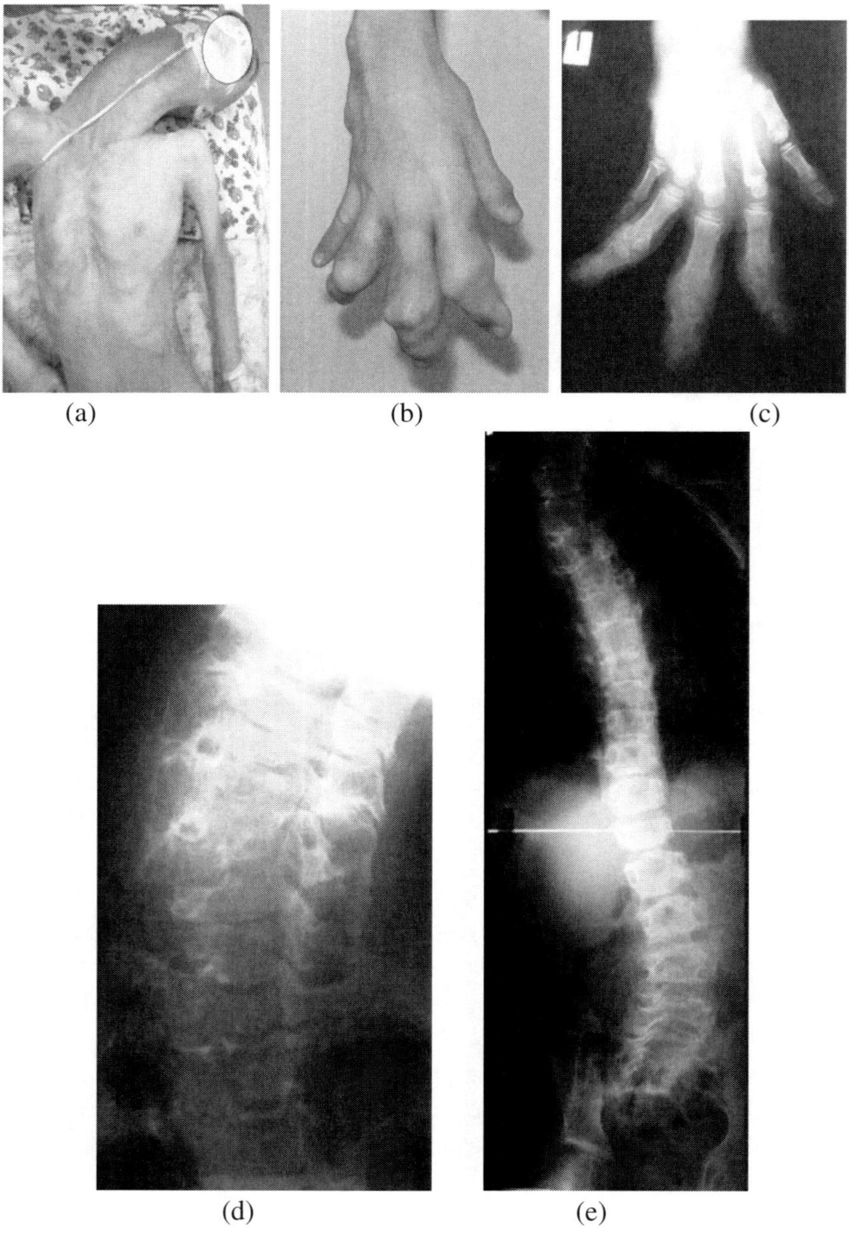

Figure 44. (Continued).

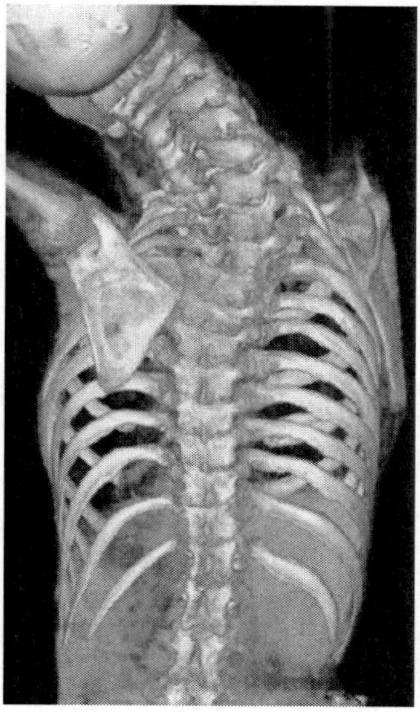

(f)

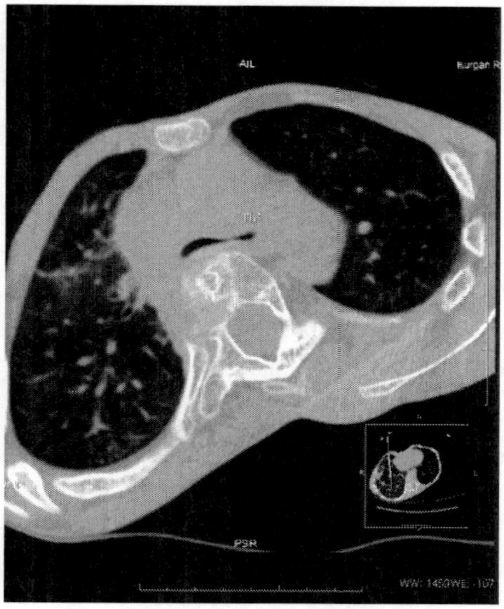

(g)

Figure 44. Image and data of X-ray investigation of the 11-year-old patient: photo of the patient in the intensive care unit: clinical torso deformation and cachexia (a), photo and X-ray of the left hand (b), X-ray of the spine (c), CT of the neck and thorax, Volume Reformation Tomography: severe rotation of cervical vertebrae (d), CT of the thorax, axial plane: signs of pneumofibrosis (e).

X-ray investigation displayed atypical spinal deformity with the apex of the major arch at the C_6-C_7 level, absence of vertebral-medullary conflict and fibrous modifications of pulmonary tissue (Figure 44 c,d). Hospitalization to the Kurgan Ilizarov Center was recommended for additional assessment and considering possible surgical correction. Though, admission to the clinic was postponed because of viral respiratory infection. Emergency admission to the regional children's hospital was required on August 01, 2011 for a severe condition with complaints of spitting up blood, coughing, frequent episodes of sleep apnea up to 1 min long. Probably, the VRI caused complications of respiratory insufficiency on the background of severe restrictive lung affection. Mechanical lung ventilation, antibacterial and syndrome–based therapy were performed at the intensive care unit. The reduced mechanical ventilation parameters led to higher levels of hypercapnia.

The boy was examined by a team of spinal surgeons of the Kurgan Ilizarov Centre on August 05, 2011. Considering his severe syndrome of respiratory insufficiency on the background of significant decompensated scoliotic deformity, it was decided to correct the deformity by halo–pelvic device as the less invasive, simple and adequate method for stabilization of the patient's condition. External fixation device was applied for halo–pelvic traction on August 05, 2011. The frame was set up in the distraction mode of 6 cm to correct spinal deformity and create favorable conditions for lung excursion (Figure 45). The surgery lasted 35 minutes. The volume of blood loss was up to 20 ml. Saturation normalized within 24 postoperative hours. However, tracheostomy was performed due to progression of respiratory failure on August 16, 2011. The patient's condition stabilized and he was transferred to autonomous breathing with *tracheostomy* in 2 days and transported to a somatic department in 7 days (on August 25, 2011).

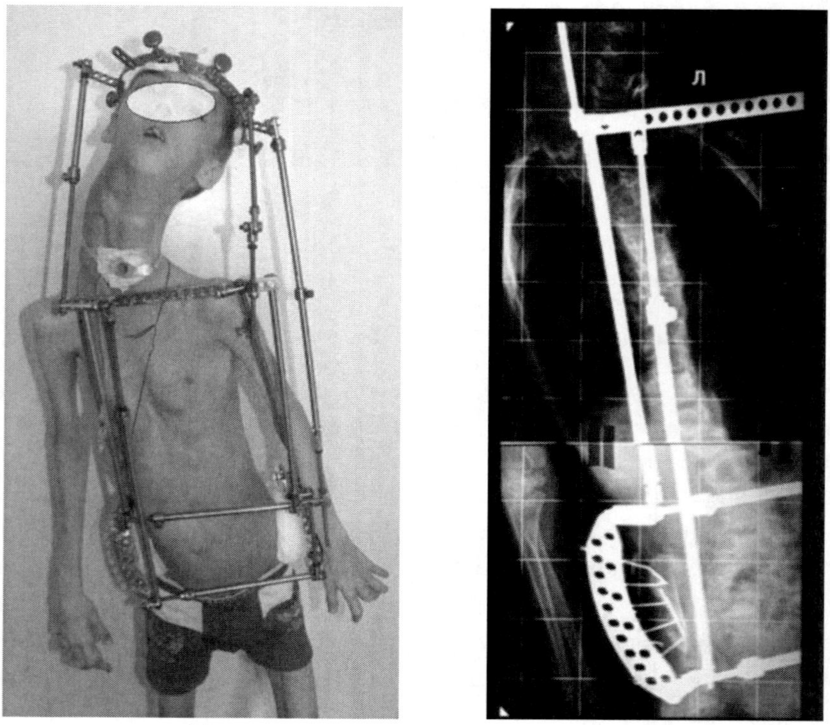

(a) (b)

Figure 45. Photo (a) and X-ray of the spine (b) of the 11-year-old patient after deformity correction with the halo-pelvic system using the Ilizarov set components.

The patient was referred from the regional children hospital to neurosurgery department of FSBI "Russian Ilizarov Scientific Centre "Restorative Traumatology and Orthopaedics" on September 27, 2011. The diagnosis on admission indicated the Ollier disease with multiple deformities

of axial skeleton, severe combined scoliosis with underlying systemic pathology and disturbed cervical spine formation, progressing muscular dystrophy, pneumofibrosis of the right lung, myocardiodystrophy, grade 3 cachexia, tracheostomy, condition after frame application for halo-pelvic traction.

On admission to the Centre the patient was able to stand independently for 10 minutes and walk with a support for 6 minutes without respiratory imbalance, and he needed help with his meals and getting up. His torso balance improved in the coronal plane with persisted decompensation, but sagittal balance was compensated (Figure 45a). Deformity correction in the frame was observed at the level of major cervical-thoracic arch up to 32° (-31°), at the level of minor lumber arch - 10° (-2°) (Figure 45b). Spirometry revealed decrease of lung capacity to 43%.

Operative intervention performed on September 29, 2011 included correction and multi-support instrumentation fixation of C_2-Th_9 segments with combined connector-type system, posterior local spondylodesis, dismantling halo-pelvic traction system (Figure 43). Loss of blood volume was 200 ml (5% of the total blood volume).

Satisfactory functional and cosmetic effect was obtained (Figure 46). Functional result assessed in a month after the surgery showed increased vital capacity of 56% according to spirometry findings and improved respiratory function with pulmonary stress test. The patient could walk with a support during 30 minutes without respiratory imbalance, eat food and stand up by himself, with torso balance in the coronal and sagittal planes being compensated (Figure 39a). The patient's weight was 21 kg (+3 kg). Checkup radiographs showed adequate screw position, spinal deformity correction achieved at the level of major cervicothoracic curve to 12° (-51°), at the level of accompanying lumbar arch to 10° (-2°) (Figure 46b). Therefore, the spinal correction was 81% and 17%, correspondingly. Neurologic assessment demonstrated positive dynamics in improving lower extremity muscular strength graded 4. The child was discharged on November 04, 2011 in 95 days after urgent hospitalization, and tracheostomy was removed on November 23, 2011.

This case demonstrates capacity of surgical orthopedic care, aimed to stabilize functional condition of the child and to improve his life quality. Absolute indications for the surgery were life threatening disorders caused by scoliosis. The halo-pelvic device was chosen because of its features as minimal surgical aggression, gradual distraction and neurologic control. Besides, we always consider this method as the method of choice for patients with severe deformities in life threatening conditions as demonstrated in the previous case. When somatic status is stabilized, the spinal departments sre fixated with posterior internal multi-support system. This strategy is substantiated by severe functional disorders, related to major disease as well as to spinal deformity and high risk of neurologic and vital complications caused by its correction.

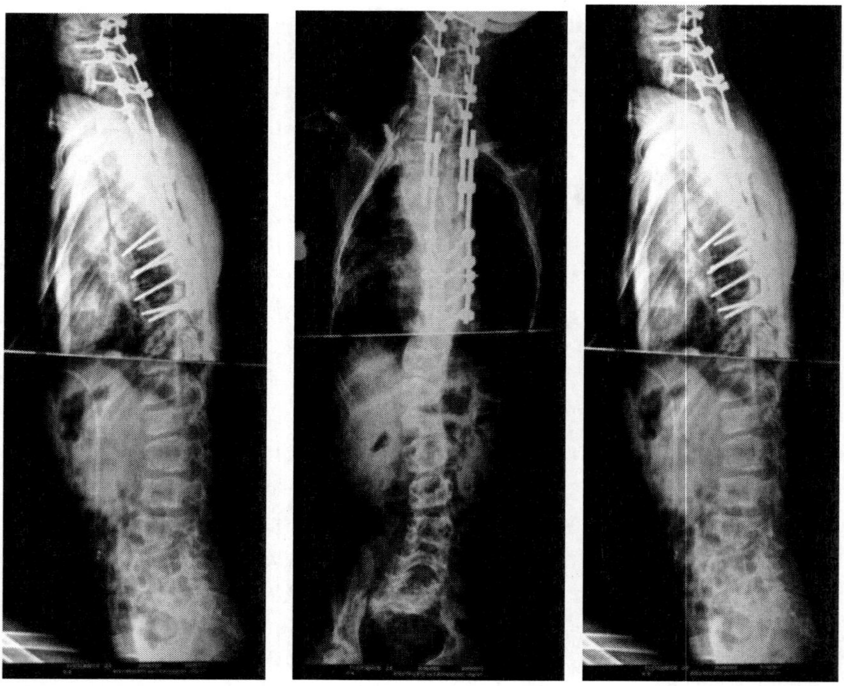

(a) (b) (c)

Figure 46. Photo (a) and radiographs (b, c) of the patient prior to discharge. Major arch of the deformity corrected to 12°.

Method of 4-staged correction are performed in two surgeries. The first surgery is anterior multilevel vertebrotomy, formation of interbody spondylodesis, closed osteosynthesis with external transpedicular fixator. The second surgery is Smith-Petersen osteotomy, correction and stabilization of the deformity with a transpedicular system forming posterior spondylodesis.

Aggressiveness of this technique determines the spectrum of its application – extremely severe spinal deformities of any etiology (scoliotic deformity with Cobb angle over 100°, Aaro-Dahlborn apical torsion over 60°, mobility of the major spinal deformity curve according to functional X-rays not exceeding 5% of the initial deformity) associated with progressing functional, neurologic and static-dynamic deficiency. Potentially, indications for the surgical treatment for those patients are vital, because of dramatic impairment of functions (especially the function of external respiration – FER). Surgical interference is based on the low-invasive principal for the segment being operated as well as for the organs involved in the surgical approach. That is why posterolateral thoracotomy and transpleural approach are not used in this group of patients. It can cause lungs collapse and turn severe FER deficiency into irreversible.

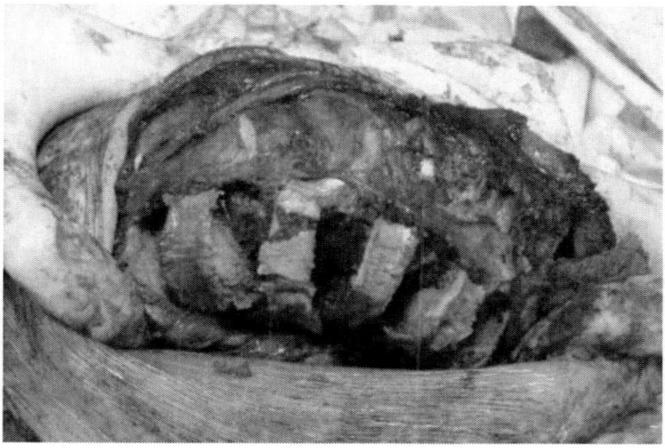

Figure 47. Apex of the major deformity arc after extensive anterior release.

The first stage is performing of an extensive anterior release at the level of 4-7 vertebrae-mobile segments of a concave side of the deformity apex, similar to anterior multilevel osteotomy at 270°. It differs from a standard technique of anterior release by an incision, which is performed parallel to the major arch along the posterior axillary line. It is convenient, as a severe torsion forms "vertebral" pleural sinus with no pulmonary tissue. After exposing posterior rib complex, 5-6 rib sectors are excised from midaxillary line with exarticulation of ribs, it provides effect of mobilization by decreasing rigidity of the thorax and a cosmetic effect at the same time. Then, extrapleural or transpleural approach to the vertebral bodies is performed. It is important to exclude a direct contact with lungs. Excision of intervertebral disks and epiphyseal plates is followed by a wedge adaptive resection of apical 4-7 vertebral bodies to correct their wedge shape. Anterior and posterior longitudinal ligaments are resected with visualization of the dural sac at 4-7 levels (Figure 47).

The second stage of the first surgical session is application of the external transpedicular fixator (Figure 48). In 10-14 days by the end of correction, a posterior extensive Smith-Petersen osteotomy at the deformity apex, application of transpedicular screws are performed followed by corrective maneuvers. The procedure is ended by formation of the posterior bone-plastic spondylodesis.

Combination of external fixation methods (halo-pelvic, external transpedicular fixation device) with variants of corrective vertebrotomy (spondylectomy through the root of vertebral arch or VCR), correction and posterior instrumental fixation of the spine, 360° bone graft spondylodesis.

Indications for this technique are deformities of a severe and extremely severe degree complicated with inflammation of soft tissues (Figure 48 a,b).

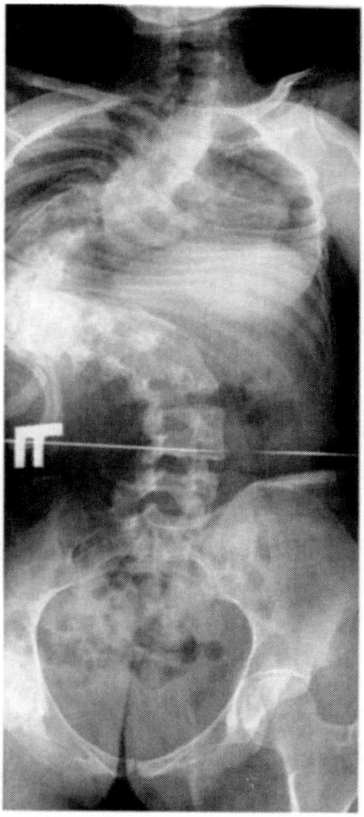

(a)

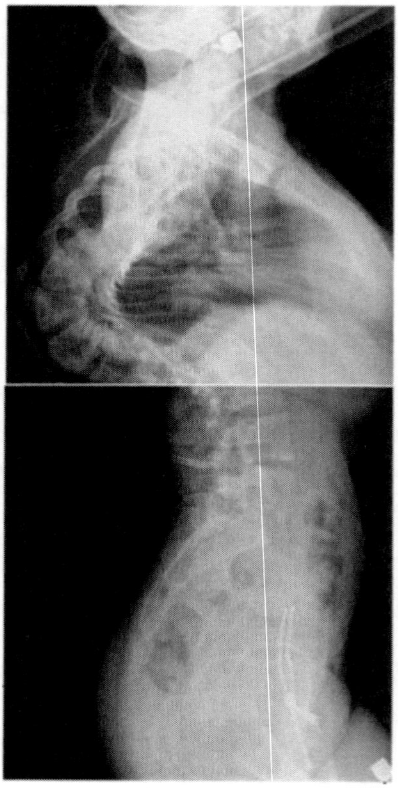

(b)

Figure 48. (Continued).

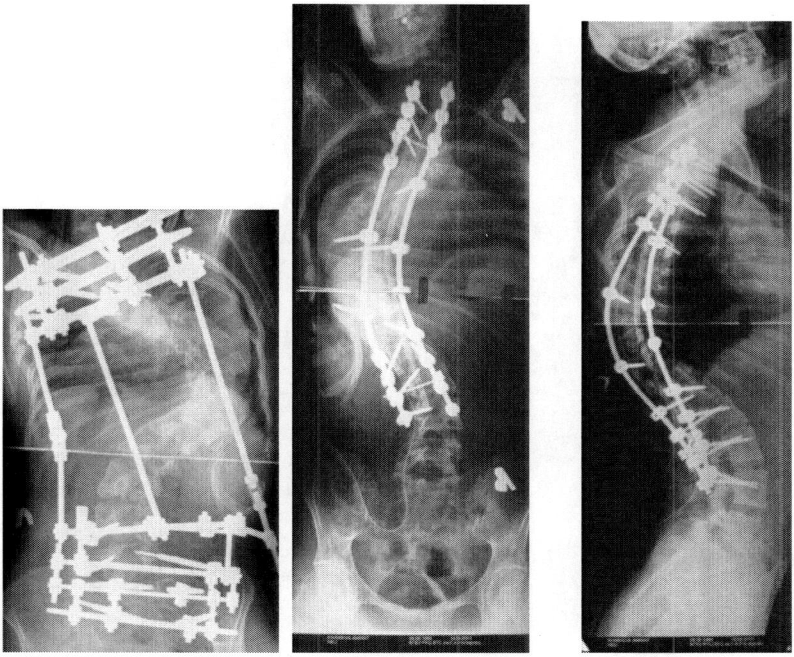

(c) (d) (e)

Figure 48. X-rays of a 14-year-old patient with typical idiopathic kyphoscoliosis of an extremely severe degree (Lenke 3C+): before treatment, scoliosis Cobb - 132°, kyphosis Cobb - 145° (a, b), in external fixator after anterior multilevel osteotomy (**c**), after removal of external transpedicular fixator, posterior extensive Smith-Petersen osteotomy at the Th_{7-11} level, correction, posterior instrumental fixation and posterior spondylodesis: scoliosis Cobb - 64°, kyphosis Cobb - 82°. Correction rate is 52% and 45% correspondingly (d, e).

The first stage is removal of implants from a dorsal approach, if necessary, wound debridement, stabilization with external fixation systems (halo-pelvic, external transpedicular fixation device, external transpedicular fixation – pelvic device) (Figure 48c, 49c) aimed to extra-focal correction stabilization of the deformity. Extra-focal external fixation provides favorable conditions for healing of soft tissues. The second stage is performed when the wound is healed. Its volume depends on the amount of deformity, its rigidity, neurologic deficiency. In our practice the second stage varied from the posterior instrumental correction and stabilization to VCR vertebrotomy (Figures 49 and 50).

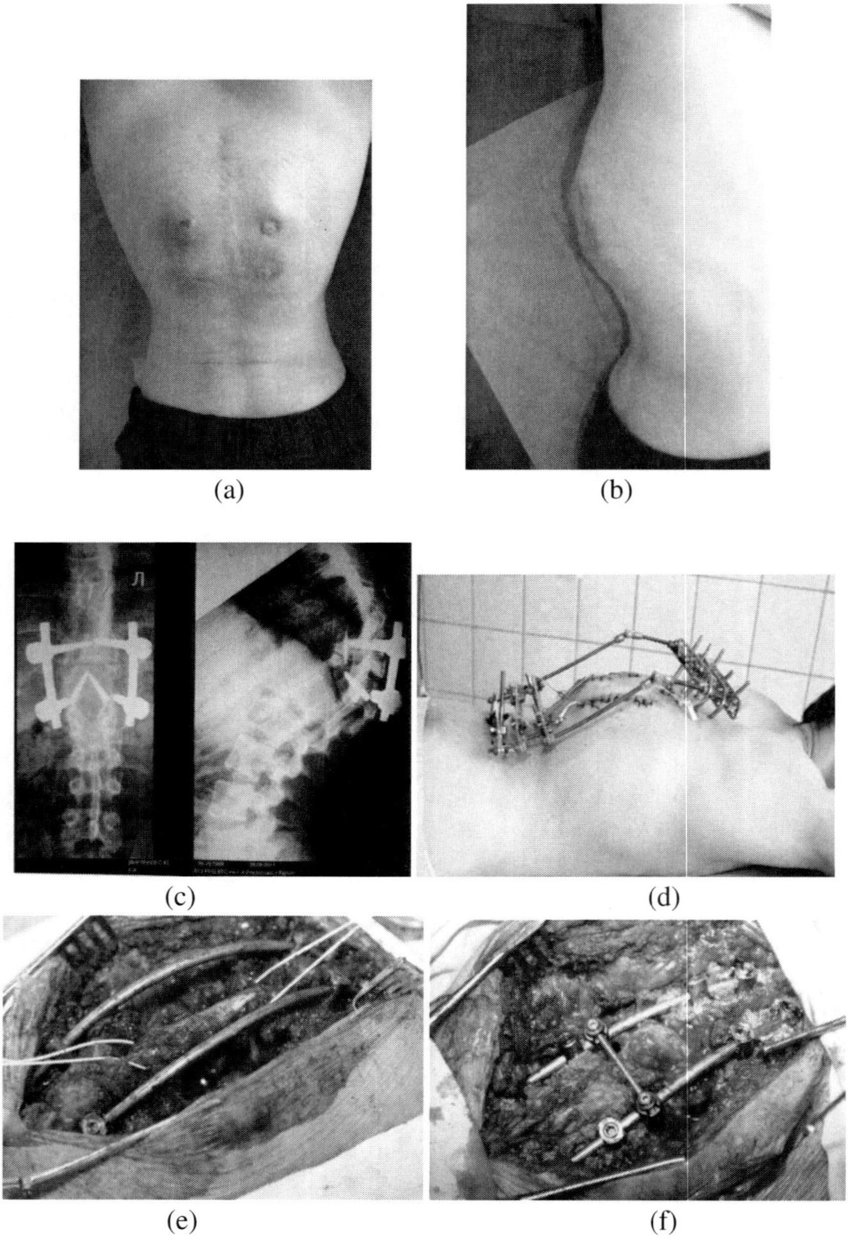

(a) (b)

(c) (d)

(e) (f)

Figure 49. (Continued).

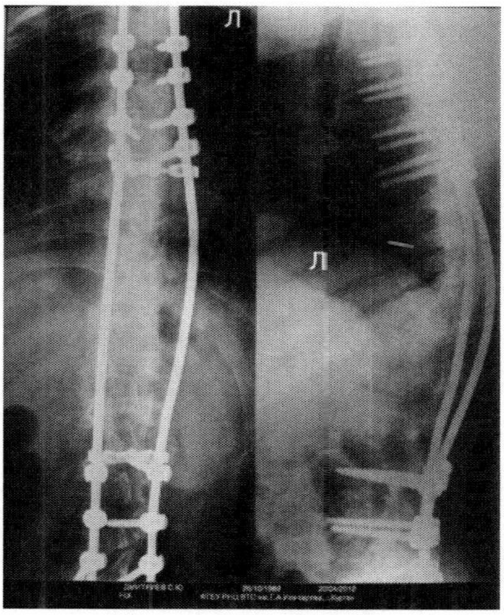

(g)

Figure 49. Photo and X-rays of a 22-year-old male patient. Spinal cord injury, late period. Sequelae of Th_{11} burst fracture-luxation with spinal cord compression. Lower spastic paraplegia. Disfunction of pelvic organs. Post-operative condition. Complications: Unstable construction. Infection of postoperative wound: patient's photo at admission (infected pressure sores in projection of screws) (a,b), X-rays at admission (**c**), Image of the patient after the 1st stage of treatment (removal of implants, wound debridement, stabilization in ExTrFix device (d), surgical steps of corrective shortening vertebrotomy with a block (e, f), X-rays after surgical treatment (g).

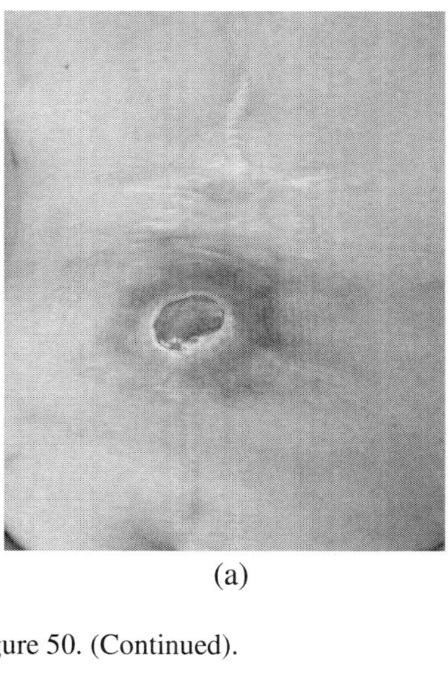

(a)

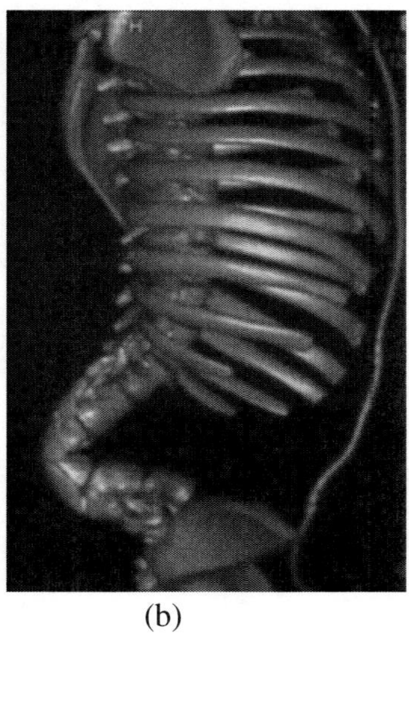

(b)

Figure 50. (Continued).

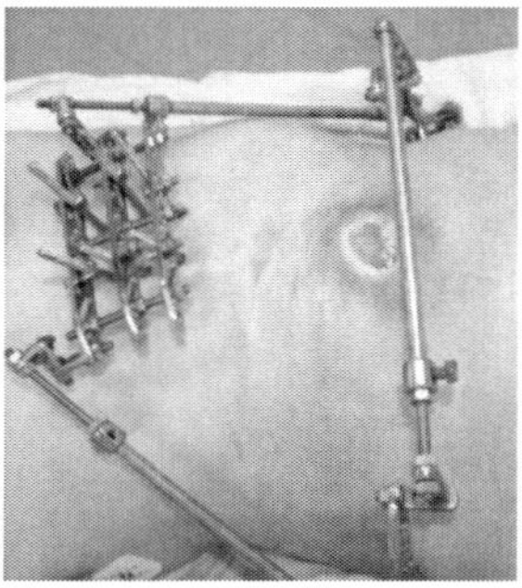

(c)

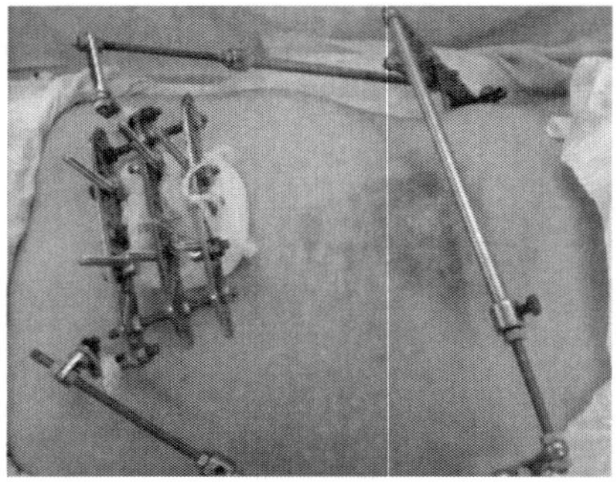

(d)

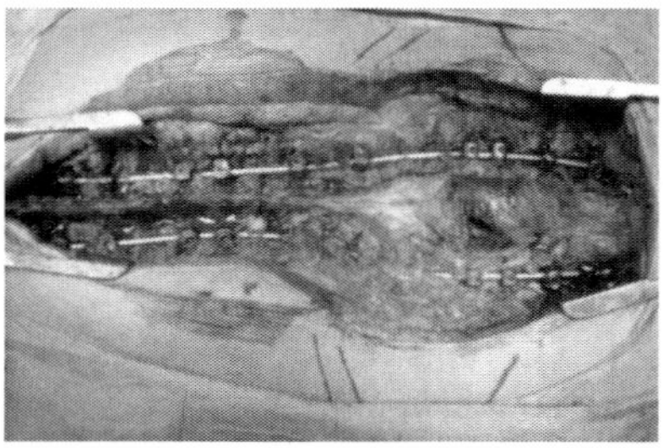

(e)

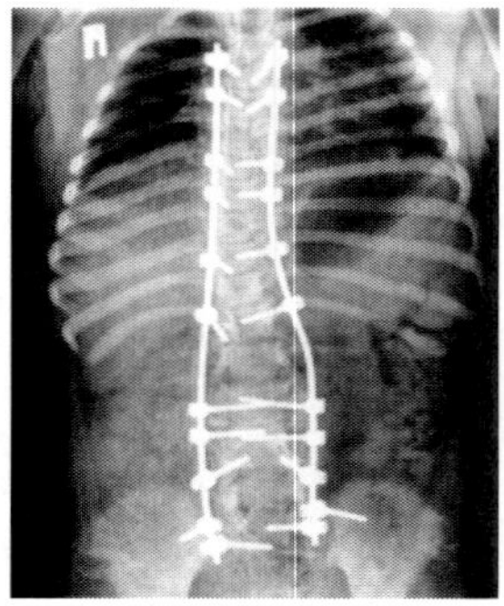

(f)

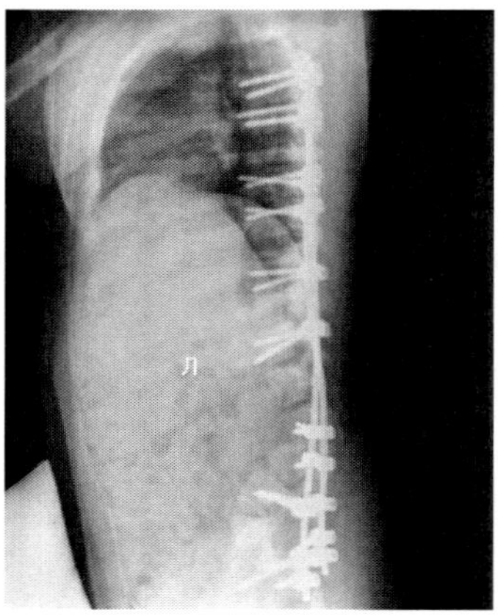

(g)

Figure 50. Photo and X-rays of a 9-year-old female patient with congenital kyphosis in myelocele with infected pressure sore at the deformity apex (a), 3D CT Volume Reformation Tomography of the spine in sagittal plane: myelodysplasia, dysraphy with hypogenesis of the posterior column and secondary structural wedge transformation of lumbar vertebral bodies (b), application of ExTrFix – pelvic device for wound healing by means of extrafocal fixation (c, d), surgery (e) and X-rays after corrective vertebrotomy and posterior instrumental fixation (f, g). Deformity correction of 84%.

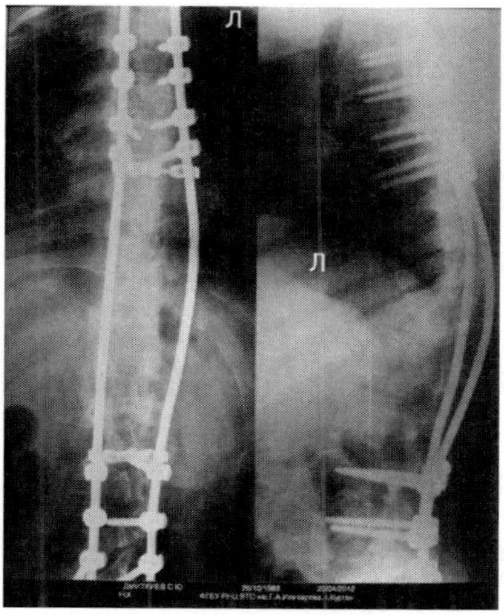

(g)

Figure 49. Photo and X-rays of a 22-year-old male patient. Spinal cord injury, late period. Sequelae of Th_{11} burst fracture-luxation with spinal cord compression. Lower spastic paraplegia. Disfunction of pelvic organs. Post-operative condition. Complications: Unstable construction. Infection of postoperative wound: patient's photo at admission (infected pressure sores in projection of screws) (a,b), X-rays at admission (**c**), Image of the patient after the 1st stage of treatment (removal of implants, wound debridement, stabilization in ExTrFix device (d), surgical steps of corrective shortening vertebrotomy with a block (e, f), X-rays after surgical treatment (g).

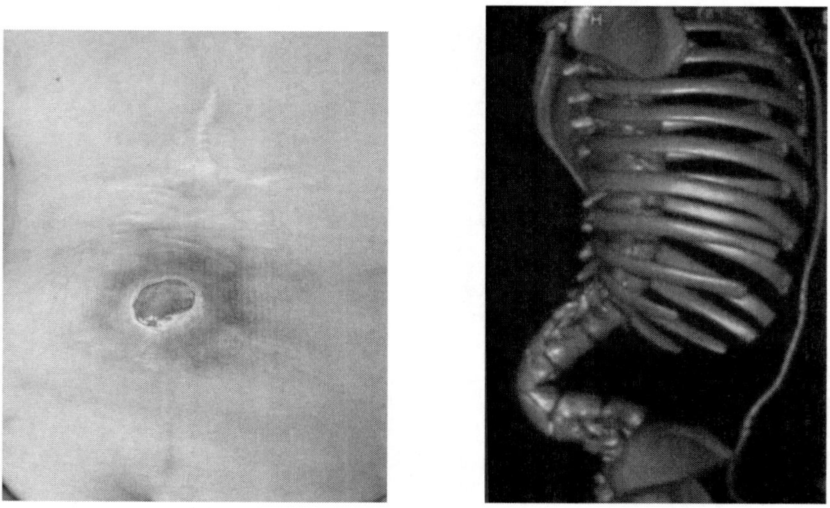

(a) (b)

Figure 50. (Continued).

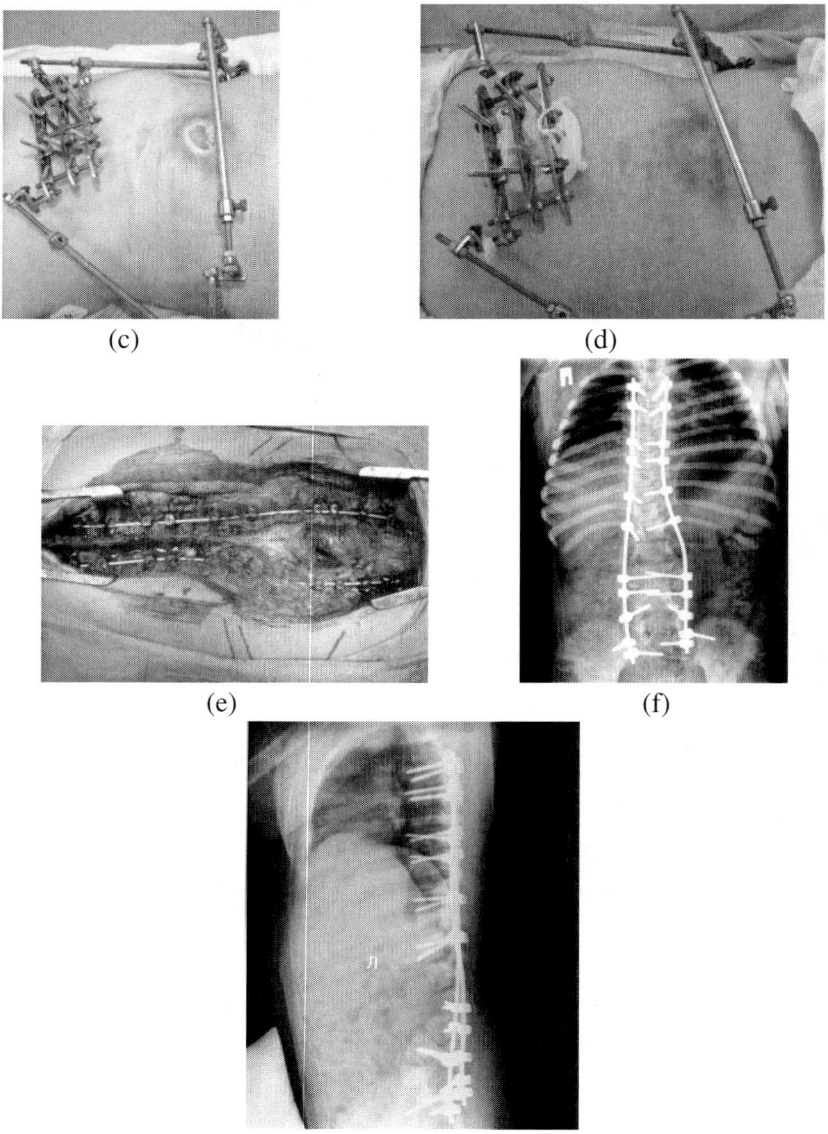

Figure 50. Photo and X-rays of a 9-year-old female patient with congenital kyphosis in myelocele with infected pressure sore at the deformity apex (a), 3D CT Volume Reformation Tomography of the spine in sagittal plane: myelodysplasia, dysraphy with hypogenesis of the posterior column and secondary structural wedge transformation of lumbar vertebral bodies (b), application of ExTrFix – pelvic device for wound healing by means of extrafocal fixation (c, d), surgery (e) and X-rays after corrective vertebrotomy and posterior instrumental fixation (f, g). Deformity correction of 84%.

RESULTS

Spinal surgery using external fixation is "a surgery of complications" as it is aimed to cure complicated process of spinal column deformities. Basic indications for use of external fixation techniques are extremely severe spinal deformities (Table VII.1) and local wound process.

Table VII.1. Influence of the deformity amount on the choice of a method of surgical treatment in scoliotic and kyphoscoliotic deformities of severe and extremely severe degree

Amount of deformity	Surgery		
	Mobilization	Correction	Fixation
70-100° * Mobile	• No • Smith-Petersen Osteotomy	Correction and Posterior Instrumental Fixation (PIF)	
70-100° * Rigid	• Anterior open or endoscopic release • Smith-Petersen Osteotomy	*Possible* Traction with ExTrFix or halo-pelvic device	PIF
Over 100° *	• Anterior multilevel osteotomy • Pedicle Subtraction Osteotomy • Vertebral Column Resection • Smith-Petersen Osteotomy	Traction with ExTrFix or halo-pelvic device	PIF

* EMG control is obligatory.

Though, analyzing the structure of complications in application of hybrid techniques, three groups can be distinguished: wound infection, implant instability and neurologic complications. Despite the external fixation, cases of wound infection in the structure of surgery of severe spinal deformities varied within the limit of 5%, which reflects average number of general surgical complications. Instability of construction, provoked by the bone resorbtion, despite its rareness was more often observed in young patients. It can be explained by bone-cartilaginous model of vertebrae and pelvis. Malposition and fracture of screws were in correlation with the scoliosis degree and torsion amount and ranged within 5-9%. Use of combined techniques in spinal deformity surgery allowed to decrease the rate of severe neurologic complications from 40% to 7%. It can be concluded that the method has average but controlled rate of complications.

Discussion

Choice of tactics for correction of the spinal deformity of a severe degree is defined by mobility of arches. If deformities are rigid in any plane, many authors recommend mobilization of anterior and posterior departments in combination with external traction [3, 4, 6, 11].

Several authors tend to use external fixators. As major advantages the authors highlight possibility of a gradual, controlled correction, both, an isolated one followed by inversion to internal fixation and an associated one combined with anterior release at the deformity apex [3, 10, 11]. Nevertheless, this method is quite demanding to a close technique of screw insertion, biomechanically substantiated design of fixator and postoperative control [1, 3, 4, 10].

Conclusion

Planning of surgical treatment of spinal deformities is very individual. If spinal deformities are complicated with soft tissue inflammation at the deformity apex or there are severe functional disorders, indications for surgical treatment should be considered as vital and hybrid treatment methods must be applied using external fixation systems stage by stage.

References

[1] Khudaev AT, Prudnikova OT, Kovalenko PI, Mushtaeva JuA (2008) Possibilities of the external transpedicular fixationin scoliotic deformity correction [in russian]. *Traumatology and Orthopaedics of Russia.* 3: 119-120.

[2] Lebedeva MN (2008) *Severe scoliotic deformities* [in russian]. Spine surgery. 4: 65-71.

[3] Ryabykh SO, Savin DM, Medvedeva SN, Gubina EB (2013) Our experience in treatment of neurogenic spinal deformities [in russian]. *Genij ortopedii.* 1: 87-92.

[4] Shevtsov VI, Khudaev AT, Kovalenko PI, Lulin SV (2004) Transosseous osteosynthesis in scoliosis [in russian]. *Spine surgery.* 2: 8-11.

[5] Wang W, Yao N, Song X, Yan Y, Wang C (2011) External spinal skeletal fixation combination with percutaneous injury vertebra bone grafting in the treatment of thoracolumbar fractures. *Spine.* 36(9):605-611.

[6] Magerl F (1982) External skeletal fixation of the lower thoracic and the lumbar spine. In: Current concepts of external fixation of fractures. *Springer Berlin Heidelberg.* pp 353-366.

[7] Kim YJ, Lenke LG, Bridwell KH, Kim KL, Steger-May K (2005) Pulmonary function in adolescent idiopathic scoliosis relative to the surgical procedure. *J Bone Joint Surg Am.* 87(7): 1534-1541.

[8] Goldberg CJ, Gillic I, Connaughton O, Moore DP, Fogarty EE, Canny GJ, Dowling FE (2003) Respiratory function and cosmesis at maturity in infantile-onset scoliosis. *Spine.* 28(20): 2397-2406.

[9] Benson ER, Thomson JD, Smith BJ, Banta JV (1998) Results and morbidity in a consecutive series of patients undergoing spinal fusion for neuromuscular scoliosis. *Spine.* 23: 2308-2317.

[10] Reyes-Sanchez A, Rosales LM, Miramontes V (2005) External fixation for dynamic correction of severe scoliosis. *Spine J.* 5: 418-426.

[11] Ryabykh SO, Gubin AV, Prudnikova OG, Kobyzev AE (2012) Treatment of combined spinal deformity in Ollier disease in a patient with abnormal verteblal formation. *Global Spine J.*1: 1-6.

In: Combined Stimulating Methods …
Editor: Dmitry Popkov

ISBN: 978-1-63483-028-7

Chapter VIII

Management of Posttraumatic Nonunions and Bone Defects by Combined Techniques (Ilizarov External Fixation and Interlocking Intramedullary Nailing). Experimental Studies and Clinical Practice

Dmitry Borzunov, PhD, MD, orthopedics*[*]*,
Alexander Mitrofanov, PhD, MD, orthopedics,
Sergey Kolchin, MD, orthopedics,
Andrey Emanov, PhD, veterinary sciences,
and Elena N. Gorbach, PhD morphology
Russian Ilizarov Scientific Center for Restorative
Traumatology and Orthopaedics,
Kurgan, Russia

[*] Corresponding author: Dmitry Borzunov, MD Russian Ilizarov Scientific Center for Restorative Traumatology and Orthopaedics 6, M. Ulianova Street, 640014 Kurgan, Russia; borzunov@bk.ru,

ABSTRACT

This chapter presents the results of an experimental study of the Ilizarov external fixation combined with intramedullary nailing in the management of long bone nonunions accompanied by anatomical shortening. These results were used in clinical practice. Combination of external fixation and nailing showed to be efficient in regenerate formation and nonunion healing in experimental settings that was proven by radiographic and histological studies. In clinical settings, such an approach to patients' rehabilitation was also efficient in achieving orthopedic goals and in reduction of in-patient treatment time.

Keywords: Bone defect, nonunion, Ilizarov apparatus, nailing

INTRODUCTION

The incidence of long bone nonunions and defects due to failed fracture repair is not high. However, these complications are a challenge for orthopedic management and patients' rehabilitation [1, 2].

Management of nonunions is based on the principles that are already known. The main principles are stable fixation and compression at the docking site of bone fragments [3].

The Ilizarov method of distraction osteogenesis that is based on the use of external fixators provided the surgeons with new ways of treating this pathology [4].

However, a long period of external fixation, the bulky size of the apparatus, pin-tract infection along wires, and the necessity of multistage operative treatment are the disadvantages of the method [3, 5, 6].

On the other hand, intramedullary nailing is considered nowadays to be an optimal osteosynthesis method for the diaphysis of long bones. The technique is low invasive, provides good stability and more comfort for early rehabilitation [7, 12].

Combining the Ilizarov external fixation and nailing allows surgeons improve patient's rehabilitation and their quality of life.

Our study was aimed at revealing the biological aspects of bone reparation and the technical advantages of combining Ilizarov external fixation and nailing. It presents experimental findings and clinical outcomes of using this combined technique for bone nonunion and defect management.

EXPERIMENTAL STUDY

Materials and Methods

A canine model was used for this experiment which was carried out on eight mongrel dogs in the age from one to four years, weighing between 14 and 25 kg and whose tibia length was from 180 to 240 mm. The experiment was performed according to the requirements of the European Convention for the Protection of Experimental Animals (1986, Strasbourg).

Bone defect of the tibia was modeled in the upper third of the tibial shaft and measured 2 cm. The nutrient artery was affected and blood supply was impaired due to the defect. The next step was the mounting of the Ilizarov apparatus which consisted of proximal and middle proximal three-quarter rings and one full distal ring with wires in each of the supports that were all connected by threaded rods (Figure 51a). The gap formed between the bone fragments due to the defect modeled was reduced gradually by daily 2-mm compression with the Ilizarov fixator during one week. When the gap had been reduced to 4 or 5 mm, fixation with the Ilizarov apparatus continued for two months in order to obtain nonunion (Figure 51 b).

Next, the Ilizarov apparatus was dismounted in order not to hinder nailing. Intramedullary nailing using the I-Loc system (BioMedtrix, USA) was performed through the entry point in the tibial plateau. Reaming of the medullary canal destructed the cartilaginous tissue at the nonunion level. After insertion, the nail was locked proximally.

The Ilizarov apparatus in the same assembly as for the nonunion model was applied again. Osteotomy of the distal fragment was performed. Compression at the nonunion level was produced. Distraction was initiated on the fifth day. The distraction rate was 0.75 mm per day made with six steps. Lengthening continued 28 days. Supportive compression at the level of the nonunion was carried out weekly. Average tibial lengthening achieved was 11.3±0.3%.

On days 7 to 10 after limb lengthening, two distal interlocking screws were inserted. Then, the external fixator was removed. The experiment was completed when radiographic consolidation was visualized (on average 45 days after completion of lengthening).

Evaluation of defect compression, nonunion, bone formation and consolidation was based on radiographic examination. Anteroposterior (AP) and lateral views were taken preoperatively, after the tibial defect was modeled, every two weeks during compression for obtaining nonunion, after osteotomy, every week during distraction, seven days after the start of fixation, and every 14 days after the external fixator removal.

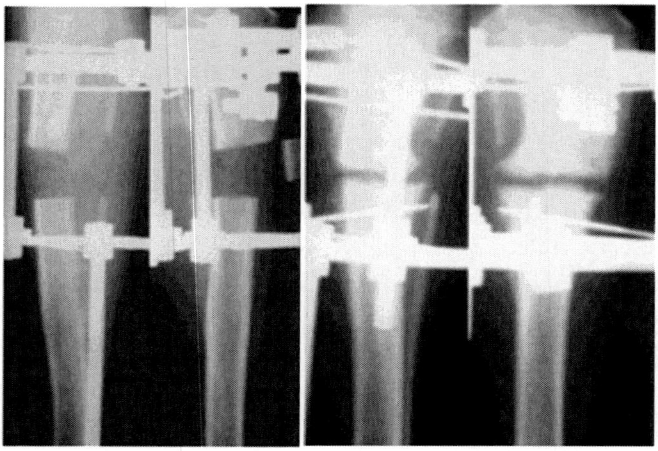

(a) (b)

Figure 51. X-ray of the tibia in anteroposterior and lateral views: a - after bone defect modeling; b - after 2 months.

Histological study was carried out with the method of light microscopy (Nikmed-5, LOMO, St. Petersburg, Russia) of celloidin histotopographic sections of the tibial regenerate callus. Microphotos were taken with the DiaMorph complex (Moscow, Russia).

All animals could bear weight on the 14th day of lengthening. There were no skin problems, implant instability or other complications. Early external fixator removal did not cause regenerated bone fracture or deformity.

Radiographic and Histological Results

The gap had inhomogeneous structure and partial closure of the medullary canal after two months (Figure 51b). The histological study confirmed the nonunion formed (Figure 52a). The interfragmentary layer contained vascularized fibrous tissue and groups of adipose cells (Figure 52b). The medullary canal of each fragment was closed by lamellar bone end plates with fibrous cartilaginous tissue on their surface (Figure 52c). The fibrous cords in the gap were united with the periosteum. They covered the bone fragments along the periphery but separated them from each other in the center (Figure 52a).

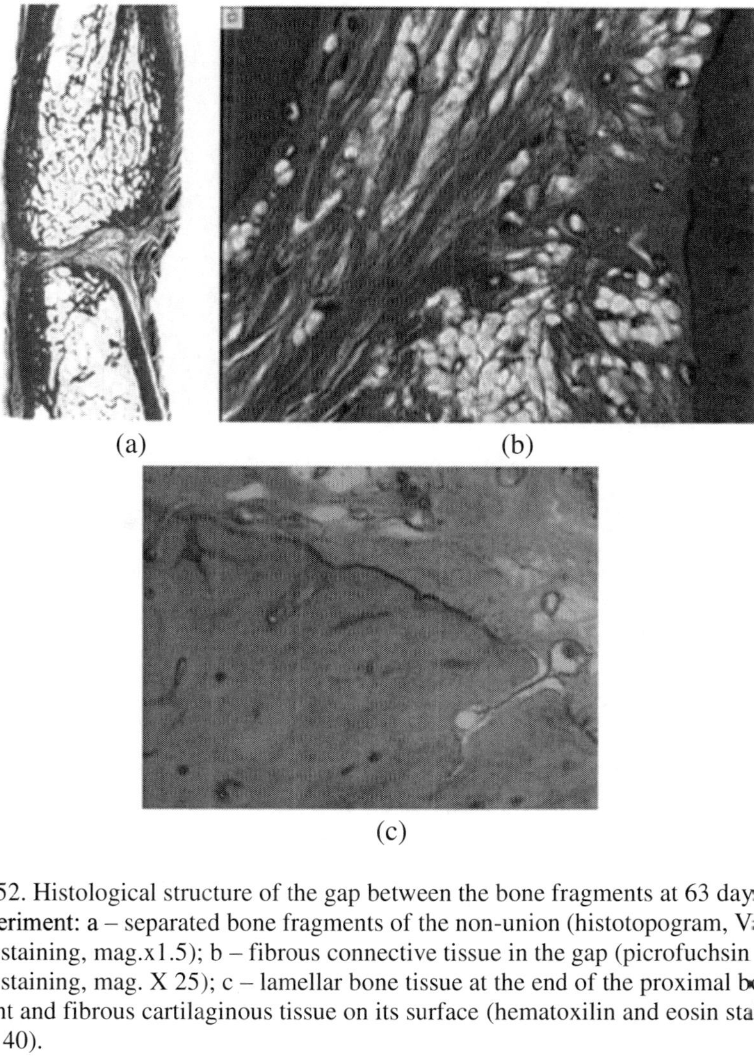

Figure 52. Histological structure of the gap between the bone fragments at 63 days of the experiment: a – separated bone fragments of the non-union (histotopogram, Van Gieson staining, mag.x1.5); b – fibrous connective tissue in the gap (picrofuchsin Van Gieson staining, mag. X 25); c – lamellar bone tissue at the end of the proximal bone fragment and fibrous cartilaginous tissue on its surface (hematoxilin and eosin staining, mag. X 40).

On day 14 of lengthening, the interfragmentary gap at the osteotomy level measured 10±0.3 mm. The diastasis at the nonunion docking site was slightly visualized. In five dogs the endosteal regenerate was 3 mm long, and the periosteal layer was 0.5 mm thick and up to 15 mm long (Figure 53a). The other three dogs had inhomogeneous regenerate structure within the nonunion diastasis. The periosteal layer was 3 mm thick (Figure 53b). Mild osteoporosis was seen in all cases.

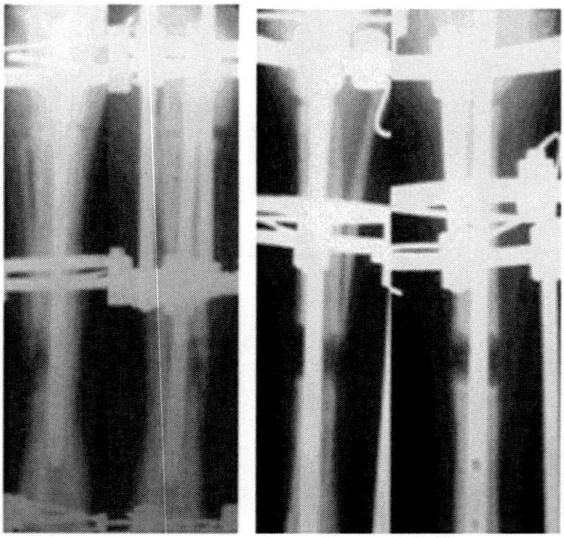

(a) (b)

Figure 53. a, b. X-rays of the tibia taken after 14 days of tibial lengthening in the conditions of combined fixation.

From day 7 to 10 after completion of distraction, remodeling of the periosteal layer at the nonunion level started in five cases. Distraction regeneration still featured inhomogeneous structure but the cortices were undergoing formation (Figure 54a).

On day 30 after completion of distraction, the nonunion healed in six cases. Fully interconnected cancellous trabeculae were formed in the distraction gap with continuous cortices (Figure 54b). Similar condition of bone regeneration in the distraction gap was revealed by day 45 after completion of distraction in other two dogs.

On day 30 after completion of distraction, the histological study of the tissue at the level of pseudoarthrosis revealed union through hypertrophic callus (Figure 55a) with cortical continuity and interconnected cancellous bone (Figure 55b). Osteoclasts were attached to the periosteal tissue and indicated bone remodeling (Figure 55c). The endosteal tissue was presented by interspersed bone tissue and vascularised reticular tissue (Figure 55d). The endosteal area had a hollow canal after nailing. The walls of this canal consisted of fibrous tissue containing capillary vessels (Figure 55e).

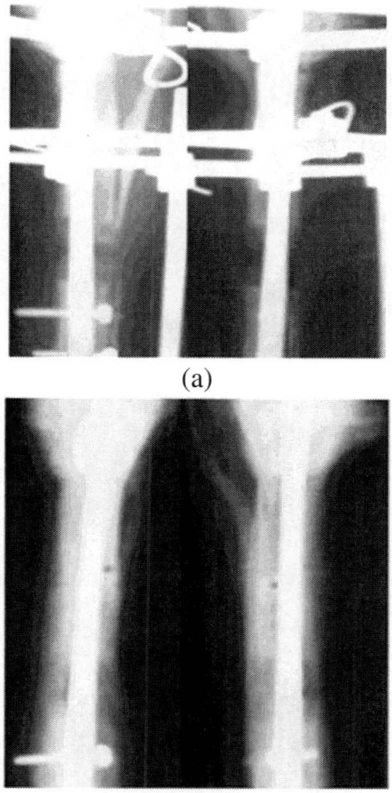

(a)

(b)

Figure 54. Fragments of x-rays of the tibia: a - combined fixation on 7th day; b - continuity of cortices all over the tibia 30 days after lengthening.

The distraction regenerate had features of a newly formed bone in the diastasis (Figure 56a). The cancellous bone tissue was in the intermediary area. The cortices were denser on the periosteal level. Bone tissue was formed of cancellous bone that contained areas of reticular tissue (Figure 56b). The periosteal callus was more pronounced on the side where the nail was closer to the cortex. On the contrary, the endosteum was more developed on the side where the cortex was at a greater distance from the implant (Figure 56a). Sinusoidal blood vessels between bone trabeculae were located both in the endosteal and periosteal tissues (Figure 56c). The medullary canal in the center was inane after nail as well as at the level of the pseudoarthrosis. The internal surfaces of the canal were presented by fibrous tissue and the external ones by trabecullar bone united with endosteal bone tissue (Figure 56d). Osteoclastic resorption was noted on the periosteal callus (Figure 56e).

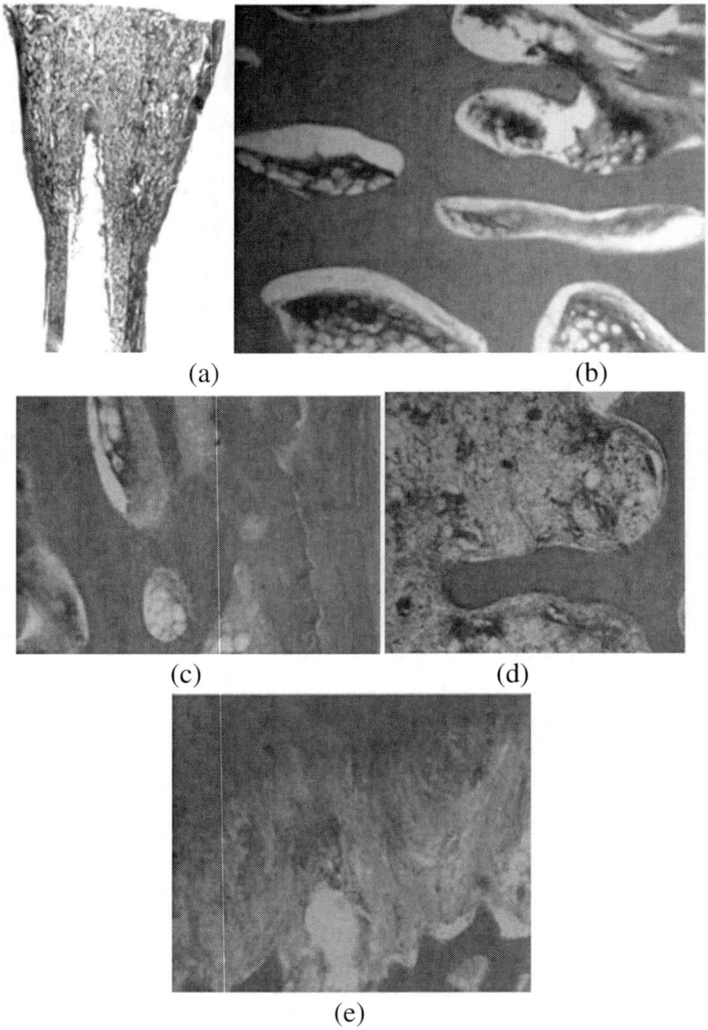

Figure 55. Morphological characteristics of the callus formed in the defect of the tibia after 30 days of lengthening: a - histotopogram of the regeneration callus; b - bone tissue part of the intermediary zone between the fragments; c - periosteal bone tissue and osteoclasts; d - reticular tissue with areas of hemopoesis ; e - a layer of vascularized loose fibrous tissue on the internal wall of the canal formed by the nail. Masson staining (a), Hematoxilin and eosin staining (b-e); mag. x1.5 (a), x25 (b), x63 (c-e).

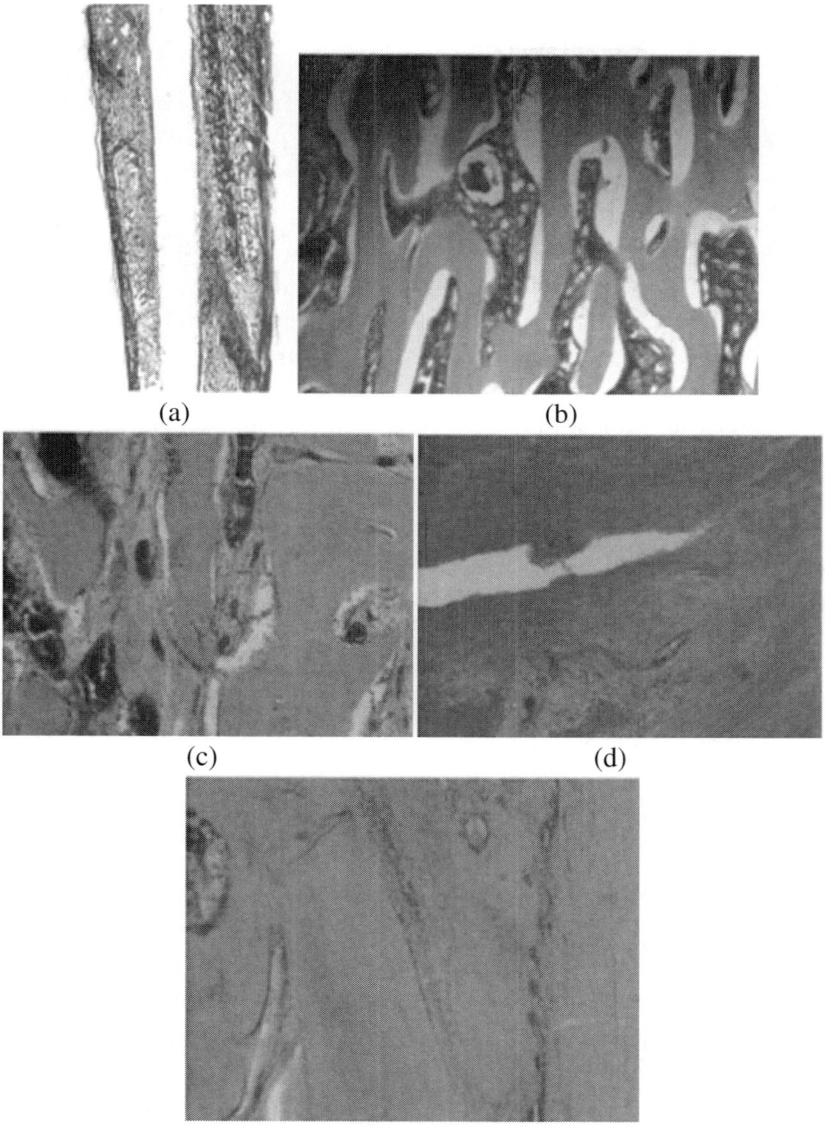

(a) (b) (c) (d) (e)

Figure 56. Histological picture of the distraction regenerate 20 days after the Ilizarov fixator was removed: a - histotopogram; b - part of cancellous bone tissue in the intermediary callus; c -reticular fibrous tissue containing capillary blood vessels with hyperemia; d - fibrous tissue; e -osteoclastic resorption on the periosteal callus. Van-Giseon staining (a), Hematoxilin and eosin staining (b-e); mag x1.5 (a), x25 (b), x63 (c-e).

Clinical Application

Combined Ilizarov External Fixation and Nailing for Nonunion Accompanied by Limb Shortening and Segmental Bone Defects

Preoperative Planning

Operative planning does not differ much from planning other orthopedic operations. It includes an accurate study of the anamnesis, careful general and local physical examination, and radiographic study. However, several issues require special attention. Evaluation of the true bone defect is a primary point because it determines the future lengthening amount to be achieved. Bone defect includes anatomical shortening as compared with the contralateral limb, interfragmentary diastasis, and the size of bone resection at the docking site (in case it is necessary). Basing on the defect assessment, the level of osteotomy, assembly of the external fixator and the distraction regenerate length are determined. The rings for the Ilizarov fixator are chosen individually. The nail of the optimal size must be prepared in view of future lengthening. Patient's preparation and anesthesia do not differ from the standard procedures before the Ilizarov osteosynthesis [8].

Surgical Technique

Step 1

The patient is positioned supine on a radiolucent table. The pelvis may be elevated with a firm cushion to make the placement of the external fixator easier. Any implant in place after previous operations should be removed in a minimally invasive manner. The entry point for nailing is produced under the control of an X-ray image intensifier (XRII). The skin incision should be minimal (two or 3 cm). Reaming of the medullary canal can be produced both with standard or rigid reamers (Figure 57). The diameter of the latter reamer type must exceed the diameter of the selected nail by 2 mm to prevent difficulties during distraction and implant instability after external fixator removal. Insertion of the nail is performed till the level of the future osteotomy under XRII control. Osteotomy is also performed under radiographic control from a small skin incision. Upon its completion, nailing is continued in the regular manner along with the insertion of static interlocking screws into the bone fragment that is to be lengthened.

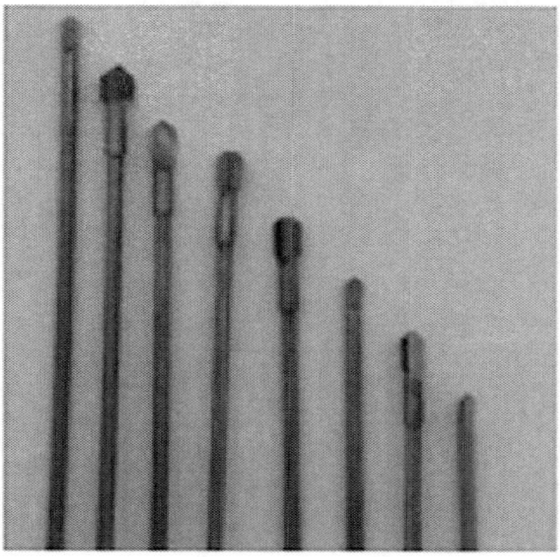

Figure 57. Rigid reaming rods. Rigid reamers may be an alternative to the standard ones in case of sclerotic obliteration of the medullary canal.

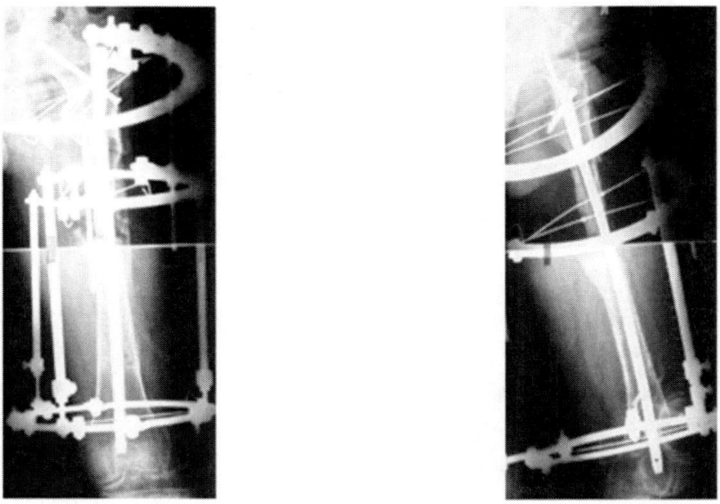

Figure 58. X-ray of the femur in anteroposterior and lateral view after step 1. Threaded rods are parallel to the bone axis and nail – optimal condition for future lengthening.

The wounds are closed in a regular manner. The insertion of wires follows. The XRII use in this case is a personal preference of the surgeon. Positioning of wires or screws is standard for each anatomical segment [9]. Wires must be drilled into the bone as far as possible from the nail to prevent possible deep infection due to skin inflammation in the postoperative period [10]. A sufficient number of wires or screws in each ring or half-ring necessary only for distraction must be inserted, as the Ilizarov fixator will be removed after lengthening. Mounting of the external fixator supports, wire fixation and their tensioning, connection of the supports with threaded rods follows. At this stage, central position of the limb axis in the frame is paramount because it determines the success of distraction in future. The operation is completed by applying aseptic dressings and radiographic control (Figure 58).

Postoperative Management and Care After Step 1

Aseptic dressings must be changed on the first postoperative day. Patient can start weight bearing and walking with crutches. On the third day after the operation, motion exercises are allowed. Distraction must start on the fifth postoperative day. The mean rate of distraction is 1 mm per day made with four steps. Radiographic checking is carried out on the tenth day of distraction. In cases when bone fragments at the nonunion docking site have contact with each other, supportive compression (1 mm every 10 days) at this level is necessary to increase stability. In our opinion, the total time with the Ilizarov fixator on the limb should not exceed one or 1.5 months for prevention of deep infection around the implant. However, if orthopedic goals require a longer external fixation period and inflammatory skin problems appear, the solution is the use of antibiotics, wire care or even the removal of problematic wires or pins.

Step 2

Full contact of bone fragments at the docking level and limb length restoration are indications for the second step (removal of the external fixator and insertion of the distal locking screws). Patient's preparation and positioning on the radiolucent table are the same as described previously. Preparation of the operation field must be very careful, especially for the external fixator. First of all, distal locking by a freehand technique must be performed. The number and positioning of screws are defined by the size of the bone fragment, nail design and surgeon's preferences. Type of fixation of the bone fragment which was transported is a specific choice for every case. Different techniques are used: plating, cerclage suture or a locking screw placed into a special hole in the nail [11]. The first and second variants make surgery more aggressive while the third one requires a specific design of the nail. Preference is given to the screw positioned in both cortices tangentionally to the nail. It makes the surgery less invasive and provides enough stability if the position of the screw is properly chosen (Figure 59).

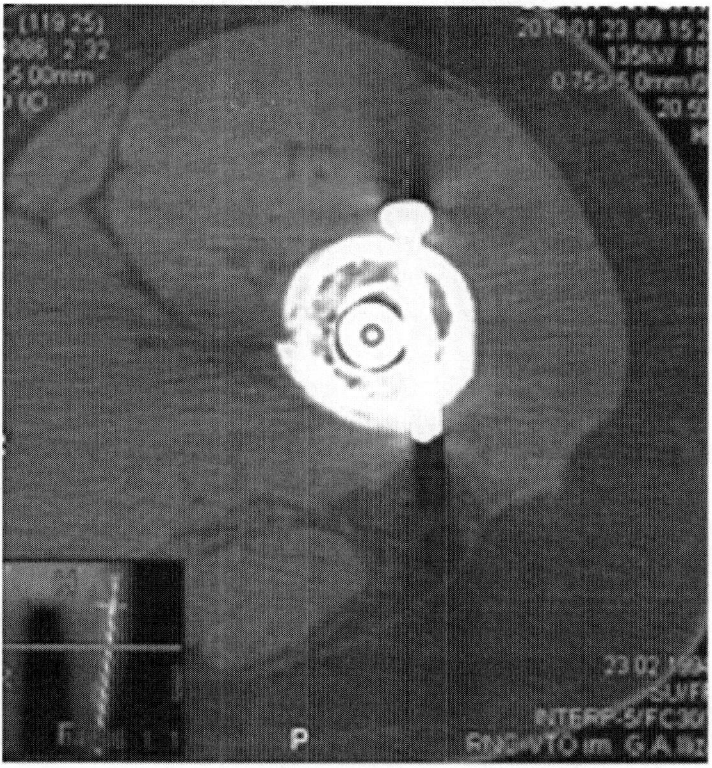

Figure 59. Fragment of the CT scan of the femur. The blocking screw inserted correctly.

Biomechanical grounding of this technique is based on that fact that prevention of the transported fragment from axial dislocation is provided by the friction forces between the screw and the nail as well as by the opposite side of the nail that contacts with the bone due to the screw [14]. When the nail is locked, the Ilizarov apparatus can be removed. Wounds are closed in a regular manner. The surgery is finished by applying aseptic dressings.

Postoperative Care After Step 2

On the first postoperative day, aseptic dressings must be changed. X-rays of the limb are taken. Patients can walk with crutches but due to static locking of the nail weight bearing is limited to 20 or 30% of the body mass, especially in obese patients. On the third day, joint motion exercises may be started. Subsequent radiographic examinations are performed in one, three, and six months. In delayed union, dynamisation of the nail is an option of choice. But it is expedient only after the distraction regenerate has fully remodeled to prevent limb shortening.

MATERIALS AND METHODS

Between 2011 and 2014, this technique was used for management of nonunions accompanied by anatomical shortening of the femur in nine patients (two females, seven males, mean age 32.75 years). In all the cases, the initial injuries were closed fractures of the femoral shaft managed with the following techniques: plating in one case (11%), interlocking nailing in four cases (44.5%), and non-interlocking nailing in four cases (44.5%). Nonunions in two patients (one after non-locking and one after interlocking nails) had been treated by reamed interlocking nailing prior to our operation, but union of the femur was not achieved. The mean time passed from the initial injury till our combined fixation was 2 years and 9 months.

Before treatment, all the patients (100%) walked with crutches and experienced pain in the femur after physical activity. The mean anatomical shortening of the limb was 3.71±0.66 cm. The mean bone loss before treatment was 7.86±1.37 % as compared with the contralateral limb.

Radiographic study before treatment showed hypertrophic nonunions of the femoral shaft. That was reason not to use any bone grafting in the nonunion area. Only reaming during nailing was used. X-rays were taken in the AP and lateral views after the first surgery (step 1), every 10 days during distraction, after the second surgery (step 2), and in the rehabilitation period (one month, three and six months after the Ilizarov fixator removal). CT was performed twice: after the Ilizarov fixator was removed and 6 months later for union verification and assessment of distraction regenerate remodeling.

The technique described above was used in all the patients. Distraction was initiated on the fifth day with the rate 1.5 mm per day in six steps, for creating tension forces at the level of the osteotomy. Once the diastasis between the bone fragments was seen on day 10, distraction was continued with the rate of 1 mm per day in four steps. During the entire period of external fixation, supportive compression at the docking site was produced with 1 or 1.5 mm in one step every 7 or 10 days.

Upon limb length equalization, the Ilizarov apparatus was removed and interlocking screws were inserted (step 2).

External fixation index (defined as the duration of external fixation in days divided by the total amount of lengthening in centimeters) and the average rate of distraction were evaluated. All the patients were available for follow-ups (6-12 months) after the external fixator had been removed.

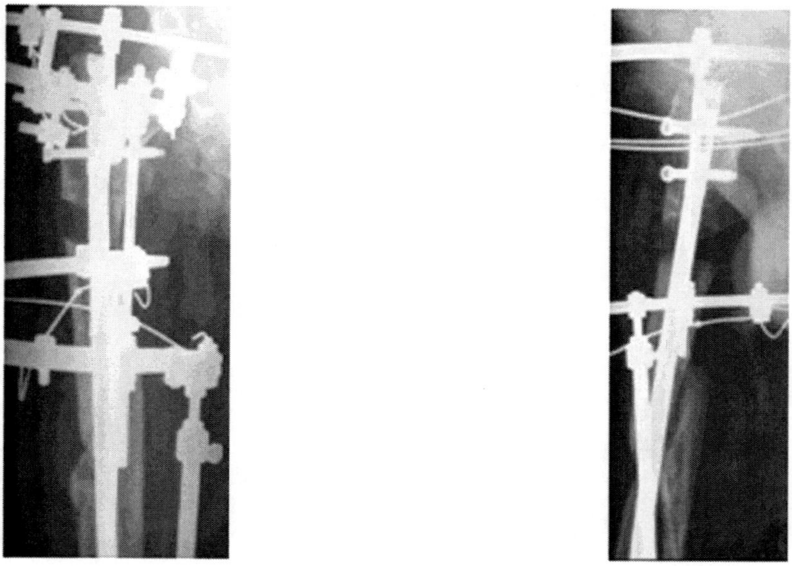

Figure 60. X-ray of the femur in anteroposterior and lateral views. 20 days of distraction. Distraction regenerate with inhomogeneous structure.

Results

On day 10 of distraction, the radiographic examination showed the diastasis that measured 10±1.5 mm in eight cases. In one case, distraction with an advanced rate (1.5 mm per day) continued for five days, and the same radiographic diastasis was achieved.

Regenerate formation was visible by day 20 of distraction. The regenerate had inhomogeneous structure, presented both by periosteal and endosteal reactions (Figure 60). CT scans after step 2 showed that the regenerated bone was continuous, had a cylindrical shape, and zonal structure. Mean bone density was 50.5±16.3 HU (Figure 61).

Mean rate of distraction was 1.25 mm per day. External fixation index was 10.2±0.78 days/cm. Such a short duration of the external fixation can be explained by the fact that the Ilizarov apparatus was used only during distraction. Fixation after lengthening continued with the nail.

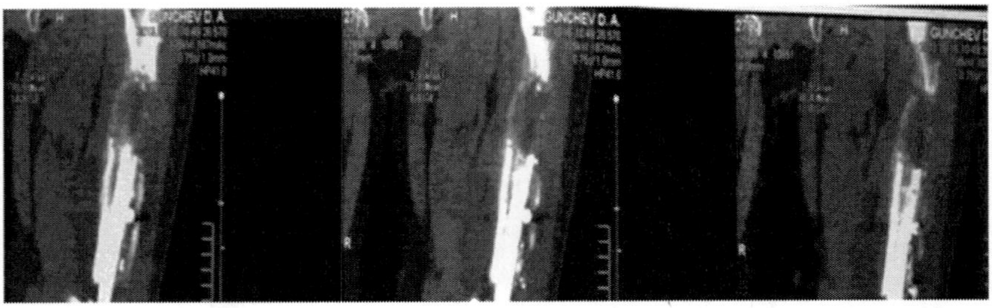

Figure 61. Fragments of the CT scan of the femur. Continuous distraction regenerate after step 2.

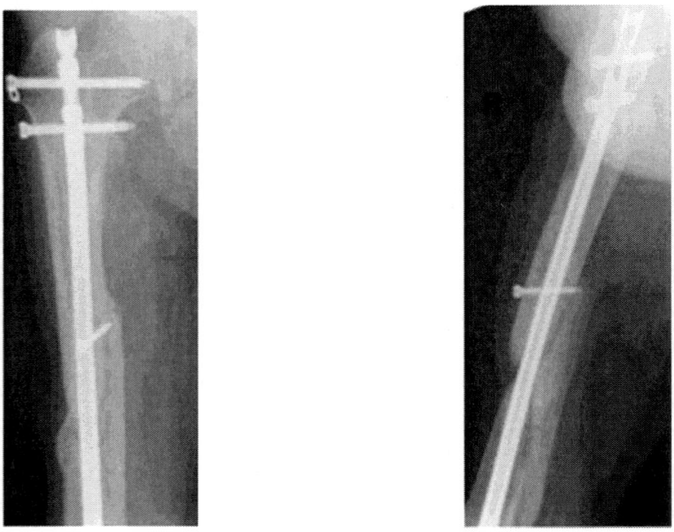

Figure 62. X-ray of the femur in anteroposterior and lateral view. Outcome in 5 months.

Inflammatory skin problems round two wires were observed in one case during distraction. Those wires were removed and new wires were inserted. Deep infection did not develop.

Combined Ilizarov external fixation and nailing allowed us to achieve restoration of the limb length in all the cases. Consolidation of the distraction regenerate was achieved within five to 6 months after the Ilizarov apparatus had been removed. Nonunion healed after five or 6 months in eight cases. On the X-rays, continuity of three or four cortices at the nonunion level and along the regenerate area was seen (Figure 62). CT scans performed at that period showed the density values of 810-950 HU on both levels.

In one case, a delayed union was diagnosed at a 6-months' follow-up. Distal interlocking screws were removed in this case, and three months later the bone united.

Instability of the nail did not develop. Once the nonunion had healed, all the patients could walk without crutches bearing full weight on the limb.

DISCUSSION

Ilizarov's contribution [4] into the management of bone nonunions and defects is considered to be one of the most important developments in the orthopedics of the XX century [3]. Distraction osteogenesis is still the main method in the treatment of the patients with large bone defects and deformities [9]. Orthopedic problems that cannot be corrected simultaneously have a chance to be eliminated by gradual distraction. However, a long postoperative period with the external fixator on the limb forced the surgeons to search for the ways to shorten that period and improve patients' quality of life.

Interlocking nailing was first described by G. Kuentscher. It has evolved to a method with biological justification and worldwide practice in fracture treatment [12].

Reaming of the medullary canal has several biologic effects. One of them is a strong hyperaemic reaction which results in revascularization of the bone cortex [13]. As the area of pseudoartrosis has a poor blood supply, this effect serves to success in nonunion treatment with nailing [7].

Analyzing all the pros and cons of external fixation and intramedullary nailing, we combined these techniques. Our experimental study has shown that the process of distraction regeneration features the typical pattern, even in the conditions of impaired blood supply.

Revascularization after reaming and nail insertion results in an expressed periosteal reaction, both in the nonunion and distraction regenerate areas. Such a periosteal reaction is a sign of adequate blood supply from the periosteum and surrounding soft tissues. It is not caused by instability between bone fragments.

In clinical settings, such an approach to nonunion treatment provided the conditions for early rehabilitation and allowed the patients to fulfill more physical activities. Moreover, external fixation period reduced, in-patient stay decreased, and postoperative recovery was faster as compared with the traditional Ilizarov method [10].

CONCLUSION

Intramedullary nailing can be used in combination with the Ilizarov external fixation for management of nonunions accompanied by limb shortening. The combined use of these two techniques allows stimulation of bone formation in the conditions of impaired blood supply. Intramedullary nailing improves the stability of the transported bone fragment and provides an opportunity to remove the Ilizarov apparatus earlier. We conclude that the combined Ilizarov external fixation and nailing is a highly efficient technique to obtain good outcomes in the management of this pathology.

REFERENCES

[1] Saleh KJ, Hak DJ, Nierengarten MB (2001) Socioeconomic burden of traumatic tibial fractures: non union or delayed union. *MedScape Orthopaedics Clinical updates*, pp 1–22.

[2] Heppenstall RB (ed) (1980) Fracture treatment and healing. WB Saunders, Philadelphia.

[3] Marti RK, Kloen P (2011) Concepts and cases in non-union treatment. AO Foundation, Switzerland.

[4] Ilizarov GA (1992) Transosseous osteosynthesis. Springer-Verlag, Heidelberg. Green SA (1984) Complications of external fixation. *AAOS Instr. Course Lect.* 33:138–143.

[5] Paley D (1991) Problems, obstacles and complications of limb lengthening. In: Bianchi Maiocchi A, Aronson J (eds) Operative principles of Ilizarov. Williams and Wilkins, Baltimore, pp 352–366.

[6] Hierholzer C, Glowalla C, Herrler M, von Rüden C, Hungerer S, Bühren V, Friederichs J (2014) Reamed intramedullary exchange nailing: treatment of choice of aseptic femoral shaft nonunion. *J. Orthop. Surg. Res.* 2014 Oct 10;9(1):88.

[7] Mazzarello F, Puncuh F, Lampugnani E et al. (1997) Limb external devices application: anesthetic procedures comparison. Gaslini 29:55–60.

[8] Solomin L (2012) The Basic Principles of External Skeletal Fixation Using the Ilizarov and Other Devices. 2nd rev. Springer, 1593 p.

[9] Paley D, Herzenberg JE, Paremain G, Bhave A (1997) Femoral lengthening over an intramedullary nail: a matched-case comparison with Ilizarov femoral lengthening. *J. Bone Joint Surg. Am.* 79(10):1464–1480.

[10] Raschke MJ, Mann JW, Oedekoven G, Claudi BF (1992) Segmental transport after undreamed intramedullary nailing/ Preliminary report of a "Monorail" system. *Clin. Orthop. Relat. Res.* 282:233-240.

[11] Vécsei V, Hajdu S, Negrin LL (2011) Intramedullary nailing in fracture treatment: history, science and Küntscher's revolutionary influence in Vienna, Austria. *Injury*. 2011 Sep;42 Suppl 4:S1-5.

[12] Klein MP, Rahn BA, Frigg R, Kessler S, Perren SM (1990) Reaming versus non-reaming in medullary nailing: interference with cortical circulation of canine tibia. *Arch. Orthop. Trauma Surg.* 109:314-316.

[13] Stedtfeld HW, Mittlmeier T, Landgraf P, Ewert A (2004) The logic and clinical applications of blocking screws. *J. Bone Joint Surg Am.* 86-A Suppl 2:17-25.

EDITOR'S CONTACT INFORMATION

Dr. Dmitry Popkov
Chief of Scientific and Clinical Laboratory
For deformity correction and limb lengthening
Russian Ilizarov Scientific Center
for Restorative Traumatology and Orthopaedics
Email: dpopkov@mail.ru

INDEX

A

B

C

D

E

F

G

H

I

L

M

N

O

P

R

S

T

U

V

W